T/

Dear Lord, the
The patients were restless and some were wired.
The call lights were numerous; too many to please.
I only wanted to put them at ease.

The look on some showed hopelessness and fear
They wanted to talk, so I stayed near
I held their hand and wiped their brow
And asked, "Can I do more, and how?"

The hard part came when at one bed I knew
A life was ending, not a thing I could do
But comfort the family and whisper a prayer
And thank the Lord that I was there.

For being there was my call
When I opted to walk those halls
To offer a smile and open my heart
Were gifts God gave me from the start

Though I may complain and whine away
You note that I decided to stay
For my rewards outshine silver or gold
A new day a new patient a new story unfolds

So Lord, don't you mind when I complain
I really don't mean to be such a pain
For nursing is my life, my love, my all
For the least of these, I obeyed your call.

Jessie Wilson, 2012

To: Joan
From: Sue

March 2014

The Diploma Nurse:
Her Shining Day,
Her Fading Touch

by

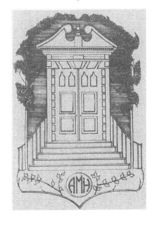

Jessie Glover Wilson

The Diploma Nurse: Her Shining Day, Her Fading Touch

Editing, and Cover and Book Design by Mary C. Findley

Cover and title page "Smith Building Door Image" from Historical Highlights of Alton Memorial Hospital and Alton Memorial School of Nursing by Rosalee Early Johnson.

Images contained in the text are credited when source is known. Image usage is included under the fair use provision of the U.S. Copyright Law. They are small versions of historical subjects used only to enrich a personal memoir.

Max Lucado "splanchnology" quote is from *Grace for the Moment: A 365 Day Journaling Devotional* Thomas Nelson; 1st edition June 23, 2009. HarperCollins Christian Publishing.

Bibliography and Photo Credits appear at the end of the book.

Table of Contents

Dedication

Dedication:

I write these memoirs to salute all Diploma Nurses, but especially to the first class of nursing students that I taught at the Alton Memorial Hospital, (AMH), namely the class of 1953. That was the first class I had the privilege of teaching, but I will always cherish the memories and the special place I have in my heart for all twenty-six classes of student nurses, male or female. They were a gift to my life and I trust my life was a gift to them.

Here is a letter I received in 1980.

April 6, 1980

Dear Mrs. Wilson,

I felt a very special need to say something to you personally. You see, I like you very much. I am going to miss you.

I hope you knew how much you mean to your teachers and students. I can see the love in their faces and feel their loss in my own heart. To us, you are special. A gal would have to be special to put up with the worries, keep things going as smooth as possible, make the decisions, fulfill the obligations, and still have time to endear herself to everyone as you have.

Do you know your particular brand of humor has helped us over some rough places during the past two years? Do you know how welcome you made us feel when we started? Do you know how much courage you've given us? I doubt that you are aware of it, but it's true.

I couldn't say it without crying but thank you for helping me to realize a dream. Thank you for caring about us. Thank you for being a warm, considerate, loving, and caring person.

I'll never forget you. I have an Aunt who lives in Quincy. If I'm ever there and have a chance, believe me, I'll look you up.

I hope you'll be proud of all of us in the future. We're proud of you and wish you the best of everything in the future.

With Love and Affection,

Johnnie Lasswell, S.N.

April 26, 1980

Dear Mrs. Wilson,

I felt a very special need to say something to you personally. You see, I like you very much. I am going to miss you.

I hope you know how much you mean to your teachers and students. I can see the love in their faces and feel their loss in my own heart. To us, you are special. A gal would have to be special to put up with the worries, keep things going as smooth as possible, make the decisions, fulfill the obligations, and still have time to endear herself to everyone as you have.

Do you know how your particular brand of humor has helped us over some rough places during the past 2 years? Do you know how welcome you made us feel when we started? Do you know how much courage you've given us? I doubt that you are aware of it; but, it's true.

I couldn't say it without crying, but thank you for helping me to realize a dream. Thank you for caring about us. Thank you for being a warm, understanding, considerate, loving, and caring person.

I'll never forget you. I have an Aunt who lives in Quincy. If I'm ever there and have a chance, believe me, I'll look you up.

I hope you'll be proud of all of us in the future. We're proud of you and wish you the best of everything in the future.

With love and affection,

Johnnie Lasswell, S.N.

I received another letter in November, 2012, from a student whom I taught in 1983:

November 13, 2012

Jessie, So good to see your precious face, even if only on FB. I am never on here, but Chuck posted pics of a fun family weekend spent celebrating his parents' seventy-fifth birthdays in Memphis, TN. Then he told me you had posted something in response so I wanted to get in touch. I think of you so often and even quote you when teaching Leadership and Psych. Does this sound familiar? "The hallmark of a professional is to know one's limits and function within them."? I use that one every semester.

I also tried to channel you frequently when I was the coordinator for a couple of years. Now I have stepped back into a straight teaching role while I am working on my DNP at Mizzou in Family Mental Health Nursing.

Your influence upon my nursing career has been strong. You helped me not to fear leadership or mental health, but instead draw upon the leadership of the Lord and His wisdom to provide what is needed for both student and patient success. I am glad you were my teacher and my program director. What a blessing!

Karin Baughman

The 23rd Psalm

The Lord is my shepherd;
I shall not want.
He makes me to lie down
In green pastures; He leads me
beside the still waters.
He restores my soul;
He leads me in the paths
of righteousness
For His Name's sake.
Yea, though I walk through the valley
of the Shadow of Death, I will fear
No evil; for you are with me;
Your rod and Your staff, they comfort me.
You prepare a table before me
In the presence of my enemies;
You anoint my head with oil;
my cup runs over.
Surely goodness and mercy
Shall follow me all the days of my life;
And I will dwell in the House of the Lord forever.

Part I Historical Perspective of the Medical and Nursing Scene of the Diploma Nurse Era

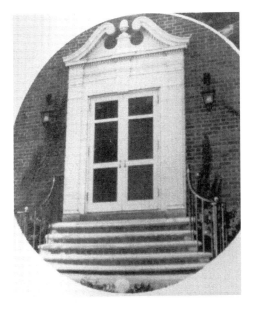

Entrance to the Alton Hospital – Author's Nursing School Yearbook Photo

The profession of nursing has within its ranks a group of nurses who have declined in number and are passing off of the scene due to natural attrition and the preference for having the Degree nurse in the modern, sophisticated health care scene. This disappearance of

the Diploma nurse will be an historic occurrence,
similar to the fading away of our World War II veterans.
Both made positive contributions to this country and
their legacy should not be forgotten. Both waged battles
and faced challenges young people should probably
never have had to face, especially those still in their
teens.

Her *shining day* took place starting in the 1940s, when we
saw the proliferation of community hospitals, until the
phasing out of these Diploma programs began in the
late sixties and seventies. I was one of these Diploma
nurses, schooled between 1947 and 1950, and had a
forty-year career in nursing practice, nursing education,
and nursing administration. I believe I am qualified to
write this story. In fact, it is a story that has been
burning in my soul for the past fifty years. I must see to
it that her story is honored and preserved.

I will do this by letting you accompany me through
three years of the life of this Diploma student nurse. In
this book you will find history, heartwarming tales,
fascinating information, and even one or two things that
will shock you. This story will endear you to this nurse.
Others might have viewed events differently from my
perceptions of these days, but this is an "insider's view",
my own story of my entry into the nursing field.

It was this Diploma nurse who provided much of the
nursing care during a strategic period after the 1930s
Depression. She worked amid limited medical resources
and technology. The drugs we have now did not exist.
Working conditions were not ideal and hard work was

often rewarded with minimal compensation. But this was shortly after the Depression. Workers' issues were just starting to be addressed and the economy was still recovering. The patients who were hospitalized were usually the critically ill. Because of the lack of intensive care units, immunizations, antibiotics, and modern technology, hands-on nursing care was crucial.

I will blend my actual experiences as a Diploma student with important aspects of the ongoing drama of the nursing history of that time. This will give the reader a historical narrative of not only the Diploma nurse, but of the other existing nursing programs; the conflict over the control and destiny of these Diploma programs; and the reason that today the nurse with a four-year degree will most likely be recognized as *the* Registered Nurse in the modern-day setting. At least that is the course being considered. It is necessary for you to understand this historical account as it related to and affected the Diploma nurse. It illustrates how her journey was made more difficult in the time in which she was schooled and in which she practiced.

Training and/or *apprenticeship* were terms used to describe the learning process, which included some science courses, nursing theory, and clinical experience. These programs were operated by the hospitals. Most programs had some liberal arts classes as well, but certainly not as much as for the Degree student. For this reason the Diploma nurse became a target for criticism, accused by some elitists of lacking social grace. I say "she" because, at the time I am focusing on, men were neither wanted nor encouraged, and at times prohibited from entering nursing. It was a woman's field. Society felt nursing was a woman's work. Men eventually, of course, were allowed to enter nursing.

The criticism of the nurse lacking social graces may have applied to the illegitimate, so-called "nursing programs" before the forties, but certainly not to the majority of the hospital programs for Diploma nurses. Please know that just passing through the doors of a college campus does not guarantee the development of social graces, either. If you ever taught, as I did, on the university campuses during the sixties and early seventies, you will know why I make this statement.

Other criticisms of this student nurse and of Diploma graduates were as follows: the student was used as "free labor", replacing the Registered Nurse, thus saving the hospital money; these nurses tolerated poor working conditions and low salaries and offered no resistance to management; and this nurse was expected to have absolute loyalty to the institutions where paternalistic authority reigned. Let us remember the times in which this nurse lived. Women in other fields were caught in the same climate, and faced similar work-related issues.

As you read bits of nursing history, it becomes quite obvious that there was no love lost between the nursing leaders and the hospital administrators. A philosophical divide existed in this country as to the management of health care. Nursing accused hospitals of being big money-making businesses. It is interesting that this same issue is being fought over today. Name-calling continues between these two ideologies. Today the one side calls the other side anarchist and the other side is called socialist. The hospitals were referred to as slave masters of their employees back then. Seems as if things have not changed, have they?

In spite of the controversy and conflict surrounding the nurse from these programs, society, in my opinion, was blessed to have been cared for by such a nurse. This nurse did have the skills and knowledge to have functioned so well these sixty-plus years. How is it even conceivable that this nurse's educational program was considered sub-par by some, yet its graduates have survived on the front lines of health care all of these years with a lasting touch of grace, knowledge, and skill?

There were three other nursing programs that existed or came on the scene as well: the twelve-to-eighteen-month Licensed Practical Nurse; the two-year Associate Degree Nurse; and the Bachelor of Science completion program. The country already had the four-to-five-year degree nursing programs but these were not feasible for the average young woman at this time. I had the privilege later in my career of implementing and directing an Associate Degree Nursing program (A.D.N.) and a B.S.N. completion program, and was proud of my graduates, even though one major weakness, in my opinion, still exists in these programs.

The two-year Associate Degree program, appearing on the scene after mid-century, is a misnomer, because it was and is almost impossible for the average student to do the coursework and the clinical time required in two

years. Most of these students are working and/or
married and have other responsibilities. So for the
majority of these students it was and is a three-year
program. These A.D. programs really replaced the
Diploma nurse programs. Clinical preparation the night
before the Clinical Day was and is spent laboring over
intensive nursing care plans requiring hours of research
and writing. With work hours, class hours, clinical
hours, and family duties, the hours these students put in
are probably no less than those we Diploma students
put in per week. As much as the Diploma nurse was
thought to be over-worked, we in nursing education
pushed these students as well. I have a feeling the
students are still pushed today.

The four-year degree programs, having more hours in
the liberal arts and science courses than the Diploma
programs, lacked, and still do, in my opinion, the clinical
time that was found in the Diploma programs. The
Diploma nurse put in thirty to forty hours a week of
clinical time, eleven months a year, for three years, but
the degree students today get usually sixteen hours per
week for four semesters. The difference resulted in the
Diploma nurse being more skilled, ready to go out into
the hospitals as a graduate nurse, more proficient in
executing technical skills. The new degree graduate must
have time and further supervision to become clinically
proficient. Some hospitals have excellent internship or
orientation programs; however, not all hospitals have
such programs. This young novice is at the mercy of the
medical center that has employed her.

Graduates of the Associate and Bachelor of Science Degree programs, and the Diploma nurse programs, all took the same state nursing board exams. This gave each of these graduates the same Registered Nurse status; however, with the modern nursing student wanting a degree education, these three-year Diploma programs exited the scene, became associated with a junior college, and produced an Associate Degree nurse. The fact that I do not focus on the Bachelor of Science Degree program or the Licensed Practical Nurse program does not mean I discount or belittle their existence or contribution, but this story is about the Diploma nurse.

My focus will be on the time period when this Diploma nurse was schooled in a pre-high-tech era when television, mobile phones, calculators, computers, monitoring devices, and disposable equipment were not on the scene. Antibiotics and immunizations were just becoming available to treat or prevent infections and contagious diseases (including diphtheria, polio, tuberculosis, and the other common childhood diseases). Without specific drugs and appropriate methods of treatment for these illnesses, the medical and nursing personnel were confronted with challenges not seen today. Mental illness patients were cared for in locked mental institutions, lacking the more appropriate drugs and modes of treatment we have today.

This Diploma nurse often cared for contagious disease patients at a risk to her own health and physical safety and under most trying conditions. Often, it was her touch that made the difference between life and death in her patients, and this is not an exaggeration or over-dramatization of her role. By *touch* I mean the intellect, spirit, body, and soul of this nurse, the elements that make up the "art of nursing".

Under the unique conditions of this pre-technology era, there was a need for a unique nurse. After all, the parents of this generation of nurses were called "the greatest generation" and, presumptuously perhaps, we can only surmise that this young nurse inherited some of her parents' attributes. Whatever quality they had, these ordinary young women performed extraordinarily.

As already mentioned, we gave nursing care to patients with conditions not seen today, working conditions not allowed today, with limited medical resources, and high expectations for the outcomes. Yet, this fading older generation of nurses will staunchly proclaim that these conditions made us who we were as nurses.

The war had brought new medical technology which helped to advance the business of health care, and most of all to improve the health of our citizens. We had an increase in the growth of smaller community hospitals across the country, causing a greater demand for nurses. Nursing was considered the main product of the hospital. Where, then, would hospitals obtain the number of nurses that would be required? Most of the legitimate nursing education programs at the time were located in the larger cities, including senior colleges, universities, and the large urban medical centers. The smaller communities naturally looked for a way to educate the women of their community to become nurses.

Thus, in the 1940s, these community hospitals increased their efforts to recruit young women for their three-year Diploma nurse training programs. The hospital administrators, in order to lessen the criticism of these programs, added more classwork and employed nursing instructors, as the nursing leaders had recommended. These steps were necessary to better the nurse's knowledge of diseases and nursing theory. While the nursing profession desired to have full control of these programs, the hospital administrators and physicians disagreed and, as men, they were in the more powerful position in that era.

The two nursing organizations, the American Nurses Association and the National League of Nursing, had their own conflicts. Had they united with one voice, history might have been different. So we did not help our cause. Furthermore, physicians did not want nurses to gain independence. It was a threat to their profession. This all seems ludicrous today, does is not? I do not want to make this book about the sexism of that day or the conflict between medical institutions and nursing, but it was part of nursing history and women's history so it cannot be ignored. Whenever some do not feel they are equal or that they lack the same respect and rights as others, not only are they not free, as someone once said, no one is free and all are victims. But that is another story.

It was not until the early forties that nursing gradually began to gain control of the standards for nursing education. Many of the Diploma programs did attempt to upgrade their standards and it was these programs which eventually either received accreditation from the National League of Nursing Education or closed their programs. It is these Diploma graduates from that era until well past the mid-century that I want to honor. Some are still practicing, although the numbers have dwindled considerably.

Since our nation was recovering from the Great Depression, a college education was not feasible for the average young woman. This was due to economics and the physical distances of these schools from the smaller communities. I, for one, along with hundreds of other young women, would *never* have had an opportunity to become a nurse and build a very productive career for the next forty years had it not been for these hospital programs. Forgive me if I seem grateful!

These programs were not the ideal in the minds of the nursing leaders, but what they wanted was not possible at that moment in history. We had a nursing shortage, for one thing, and so, to have a nursing school available was a natural outcome for a small hospital. Indeed, the goal of the nursing leaders to place all nursing education in higher educational institutions was a worthy one. But in my opinion, it was not the right time or the right climate for it to be realized. This dream was not to come to fruition until the sixties and seventies.

Movement in this direction was hastened when early in the 1950s the National League of Nursing bestowed accreditation status on the schools that met the nursing curriculum standards as designed by the NLN. Those hospital programs not accredited eventually closed or became affiliated with junior colleges or universities.

The public has always expressed pride in their doctors and nurses, but the public has not always been aware of or concerned about what these men and women have had to go through to obtain their medical and nursing education; particularly, as to the expectations placed upon these students. Were these expectations always realistic and humane for these students, resulting in safe practice for the public? No!

It was not until 1947 that all states were required to have registration of graduate nurses. They had to pass a State Board of Nursing examination to offer some protection to the public. The state of Illinois already had such registration requirements for nurses. It was not until much later that anyone challenged the many, unrealistic hours interns had to work. Such conditions could compromise patient safety and jeopardize the health of the interns.

In all honesty, the real status of many of the so-called "nursing programs" between 1900 and 1940 is not a pretty story, either. In spite of the legitimate nursing schools, other fly-by-night nursing courses came on the scene, and almost anyone could become a "nurse", because all that seemed to be desired was a sort of housekeeper. It seems unbelievable, nowadays, that nurses should not be educated. Sadly, changing the thinking of society takes time.

The fact that we were not degree nurses did not make us less professional. We did know for sure that we knew how to give tender, loving bedside care (TLC). We did not have an environment that took us away from the patient's bedside, as is commonly the case today. There was continuity of patient care. This was critical to quality care, and still is today.

We knew our patients and they knew us. We also learned how to improvise in the absence of technology that is available today. We had to be proficient in math, since prescribed drug dosages were not available in the desired dosage or pre-packaged and ready to administer. The physician prescribed intravenous orders but we had no monitoring machines to set the number of fluid drops per minute. Nor did we have the use of a calculator to perform our math, so high school Algebra served us well.

Every generation of nurses has had its challenges and stresses to face. The joys of the profession always have to be shared with the stresses imposed by the conditions in the health care system and society as a whole. The demands of the environment, technology, needed knowledge, and skills placed on the today's nurses are no less stressful than in her predecessor's day. In fact, the demands today have finally reached the stage when even the Bachelor Degree nurse needs further clinical expertise and continuing education, since we are now into the robotic age.

Nursing today has gained more professional respect, and still remains an opportunity for young men and women who are altruistically inclined to serve those who are ill or injured. To those of us who are people of faith, caring for the sick has a spiritual component which is a guiding factor in everything we do. Faith is that inner strength that motivates us, as scripture dictates, "to do unto others as we would have them do unto us". The heart still matters. A nurse's care is the outward manifestation of compassion. Compassion has to be matched by clinical competency and appropriate knowledge. Hopefully that gracious, creative touch is also part of the art of nursing.

We concede that a changing of the guard was necessary and the nursing mantle should pass on to a generation of nurses who can meet the standard for modern-day academic and clinical expertise. One day this nurse's story will also be written. But knowing how the Diploma nurse was caught in these struggles will help you understand her journey. Comparing and judging the Diploma nurse with today's student nurse is like comparing apples to oranges. Let's judge each for his or her given day.

From one who is so proud to have been one of those Diploma nurses who wore the distinguishing white cap, the symbol which identified this nurse, I give you a wonderful love story I call *The Diploma Nurse: Her Shining Day, Her Fading Touch*.

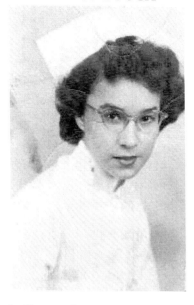

Jessie Glover Wilson Nursing School photo

Alton Memorial School of Nursing
Our Oath

We will never bring disgrace to this, our school, by any act of dishonesty or disloyalty, but will fight for the ideals of Alton Memorial Hospital, both alone and with others; We will revere and respect our school rules, and do our best to incite a like respect and reverence in those about us who are prone to annul and set them at naught; but will serve unceasingly to do our best toward school duties; Thus, in all these ways, we will transmit this school not only less but greater, better, and more beautiful than it was transmitted to us.

In Memoriam – Martha Sproule

Part II The Pride of a Community

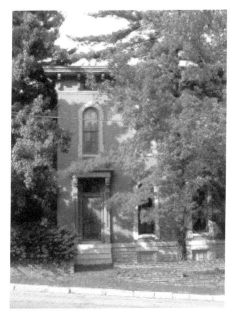

Historic House in Alton Photo by Ralph Moran, Wikimedia Commons

World War II was now over. Our citizens breathed a huge sigh. The past fifteen years had been plagued with turmoil ranging from a disastrous Depression, its aftermath, and a horrendous war. It was now a time for healing, moving forward, and facing the new challenges of a post-war period.

Our community, like others, was the face of America. The Civil War had not brought equality; unions were still young and many worker problems had yet to be addressed; and yes, religious, racial, and gender discrimination existed in all sections of the country, east or west, north or south.

People were basically good, caring and generous, but the last twenty years had been hard on families who were now focused on surviving and rebuilding and had little awareness of, or energy left for, solving huge social issues. More awareness of these issues was coming as communication technology was on the horizon to bring the world right into our living rooms by something called television.

The growth of education certainly played a major role in combating injustice and enlightening society. With peace at hand our citizens would see a brighter day in the economy and educational opportunities. We must be reminded that before the Depression only about 15% of young people graduated from high school and, fortunately for the Depression babies, the percentage of high school graduates began to accelerate.

We young women had grown up in this southern Illinois river town of Alton, Illinois. Our town was blessed by the addition of one of these new small community hospitals. We were able to enroll in the Alton Memorial Hospital School of Nursing. This school existed from 1937 until 1973, when it transferred to a junior college Associate Degree program at Lewis Community Hospital in Godfrey, Illinois. Our school was typical of most Diploma schools of this era.

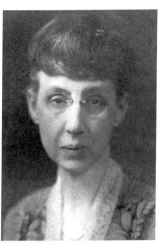

Eunice C. Smith Photo from BJC Healthcare Pinterest page Historic photos

The Alton Memorial Hospital was built on a piece of land donated by the estate of William Elliot and Alice Smith. After their deaths, two daughters, Eunice C. Smith and Alice S. Hatch, followed through with their parent's wishes, donated the land, and partially endowed the hospital under the auspices of the Methodist Church. Ground was broken in 1936 and on November 19, 1937, the hospital was opened and dedicated. One of the daughters, Eunice Smith, lived on the estate. She took a personal interest in the hospital and could be seen assisting in keeping up the beautiful grounds. She was alive while I was in school. I had the privilege of seeing her on many occasions, since she also took an interest in the nursing program. Until her health broke she sponsored a monthly tea for the students and bought each of them the well-remembered nursing cape for Christmas. She was a dignified, cultured lady who modeled poise, generosity, dignity, grace, and faith for us young women.

The hospital was a small community facility designed for 75 beds and 20 bassinets, built up on a hill, with a winding road ascending to the hospital grounds. It was well-hidden from the main road, nested in a beautiful setting of trees, flowers, and vegetation of all kinds. The front of the hospital had beautiful, white, ornate doors and ivy growing on the brick walls. It was warm and inviting, patterned after New England colonial architecture, as I recall. It is now a "state of the art" medical facility with modern buildings equipped with the latest technology. In fact, it is recognized as among the top ten hospitals in the state.

In later years, I taught at the St. Joseph Hospital Nursing Program, also located in this community. This school was operated by the Daughters of Charity. Both nursing schools were comparable in almost every way. The other hospital was St. Anthony's Hospital, operated by a hard-working group of nuns from Germany. It was a contagious disease hospital. After the relative control of communicable diseases in our country this hospital became a general hospital.

Alton was proud of its health facilities, and rightly so. Most of the same doctors were on the staff at all three hospitals. An additional hospital for this area was eventually built in a neighboring town of Wood River, Illinois. These hospitals met the needs of many rural small towns in this western part of southern Illinois. The two Alton nursing programs aided greatly in the staffing of these hospitals. These hospitals were the clinical laboratories for the Diploma students of both Alton nursing programs.

Fortunately, too, for this generation, hospitals became much more than just a place of last resort for sick people. Medical schools educated more physicians. Advances in medicine necessitated care better administered in a hospital setting than in homes. And as luck would have it, just across the Mississippi River to the west, in St. Louis, Missouri, were two of the finest medical schools in the country, Washington University and St. Louis University. Local students had easy access to these medical schools and many would return to the Alton area to practice.

This assured the Alton hospitals of having not only highly qualified medical personnel in sufficient numbers, but by operating a nursing program, the hospitals would also have their nursing staff needs met. Many of the Diploma nurses in the fifties and sixties continued their education by obtaining a Bachelor of Science in Nursing and even going beyond that and acquiring a Master's Degree in Nursing in a variety of specialty clinical areas.

These same nurses went on to take positions as Directors of Nursing Programs or Vice Presidents of Nursing care, making positive contributions to nursing education and nursing practice and leaving a lasting legacy. These are the same nurses who were criticized for letting hospitals use and abuse them in an era when, even if these conditions did exist, the chances of women changing the status quo were slim to none. At that time they may have been powerless, but not hopeless. They had faith in the future and in themselves. I cannot defend those hospitals that were guilty of such belittling practices, but certainly this was not true of all hospitals.

Rather than view themselves as abused, these young women were grateful for the educational opportunity. They realized it would enable them to enhance their lives and make positive changes in the future. They could improve conditions for those who followed them. We students and hospital employees did not feel enslaved. You see, we knew that at least our lives were better than what our mothers and grandmothers had experienced. We also believed that better things were ahead. History has proved that we were not wrong.

MEET THIS DIPLOMA STUDENT

The average young nursing student enrolling in nursing school during the 1940s was female, 18 years of age (although I was just 17), born in the late 1920's or early 1930's, and most likely Caucasian. We had all graduated from high school, while our mothers might or might not even have gone to high school. Our grandmothers probably had finished the eighth grade at most. Career choices for women were mainly teaching or secretarial positions. Our fathers had served in the recent war, and many of our mothers had covered for the men in factories. We were most likely the first generation of these families who had finished high school and even pursued further education.

Prerequisites for admission into nursing school included graduation from high school and course work in Algebra, Biology, and Latin or another foreign language. Students who took Chemistry were preferred. I had a Latin Usage course which proved very beneficial in understanding the medical terms and reading the physicians' drug orders.

These nursing students were also known as children of the Depression and of World War II veterans. They came from families who had endured hard times. They

had been raised to be respectful and responsible and
definitely to submit to authority. They knew the value of
hard work, education, and money. Most had a religious
background. All of this made these students, in my
opinion, more mature for their young age, and I might
add, more mature than the generations I taught later on
in my career. What special ingredient did they possess
that made them who they became and able to perform
as they did? As Doctor Hubert Allen, an Alton
Obstetrician, remarked 20 years later, they performed
"beyond what we should have asked of them."
Hindsight is often enlightening and humbling, isn't it?

THE PORTRAIT OF OUR RIVER CITY

We are defined by the community and era in which we
are raised. It influenced how we felt about ourselves and
life in general. The town we lived in; the schools and
churches we attended; and the prevailing local and
national cultural, social and political ideologies helped
us formulate our views of self, God, religion, values,
and also determined our biases. Positive or negative
perceptions are formed early and, right or wrong, these
become our belief system.

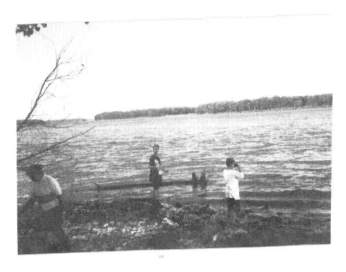

On the Mississippi – Personal Photo

This story was set along the banks of the mighty Mississippi, just below where the Missouri, Mississippi, and Illinois rivers merge for a few miles. Alton is known for many things, but probably most of all for its river, the beautiful Alton Dam, and the bridge that now crosses from the Illinois to the Missouri side. Majestic, scenic bluffs line the river. In the fall the scene is picturesque, with breathtaking red and golden leaves that attract visitors from everywhere. You can follow this scenic trail all the way up to Mark Twain's old stomping grounds in Hannibal, Missouri.

Pere Marquette Park is a beautiful resort. Quaint little river towns like Chautauqua, Elsah, and Grafton tempt travelers. Walk the streets in Grafton and go in and out of a variety of antique and craft shops. Stop in at a small cafe and have the best catfish sandwich ever. Walk

23

along the banks of "Ol' Miss" and be enthralled by the scenic beauty.

Between Grafton and Alton was a site that almost was chosen to build the Air Force Academy back in President Eisenhower's time. You know it must have been special to have been considered. The river, the bridge and dam, the hills, the scenic river bluffs, and the industrial smoke stacks defined Alton. One hill on Seventh Street was so steep that when you were at the top you could not see to the bottom until you started to go down the slope. It was great for sledding if you were brave enough to try it.

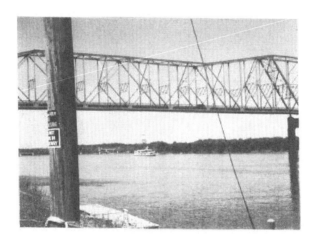

Bridge over the river – Personal Photo

The river provided great fishing. Fishermen cast out their lines and sat beside huge baskets with unbearably smelly catfish bait in them. These skilled men would mark where they had dropped their baskets by lining them up with some landmark on shore. They would return in a couple of days, throw out big iron hooks, and drag for their baskets, hook them, bring them up, and get the fish trapped inside. Beautiful Alton Lake is north of the dam and provides much pleasure for those who like boating and waterskiing.

A huge painting of the Piasa bird, based on a Native American legend, is located on one of the big hillside bluffs. I have heard various stories repeated in the river towns. Two young Indian lovers were forbidden to marry each other, so they both jumped off the cliffs into the river waters below. It was their version of Romeo and Juliet. Another version is that the eagle-like bird used to pick up young Indian boy victims. The men of a tribe decided to place a young boy in the center of a circle. They all gathered around him high up on the bluffs. As the eagle swooped down to grab the boy, the men shot arrows, trying to wound the bird under his wing, which was his "Achilles Heel". They were successful and the bird fell into the water below. I cannot verify these legends. Many stories change with retelling and acquire variations as time passes.

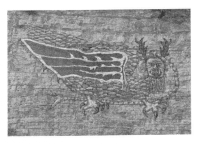

Modern Repainting of the Piasa Bird Photo by Burfalcy Creative Commons

In the middle of town is beautiful Rock Spring Park. It had trees of every kind, flowering vegetation, and a cool, sprawling brook where we kids would catch crawdads and wade during the hot summer days. It offered our citizens a restful playground and hosted many a family picnic.

A flour mill sat on the edge of downtown Alton. Farther east were other industries, huge smoke stacks, and railroads. The look was definitely industrial. Although the buildings were not very attractive, they were havens where hard-working men and women made a living to better their lives and provide for their children.

Alton is also known for its famous son, Robert Wadlow, "Alton's gentle giant", who stood 8 feet, 11.1 inches tall. As a youngster he operated a lemonade stand in his front yard on Brown Street. Robert Wadlow died in his early twenties due to an infection caused by a heel blister. In my memory, his gentleness represented the tenor of our city.

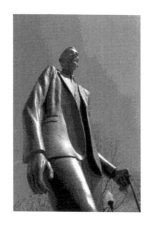

Robert Wadlow Statue Photo by Chrissy Wainwright Flikr Commons

A very realistic statue of Robert stands across from what used to be Shurtleff College, an American Baptist College, but is now a branch of Southern Illinois University. Life was simple, quiet, uncomplicated and just plain good. You see, we all knew we had a better life than our grandparents. So what we had we appreciated greatly.

Because of its industries, Alton attracted many new families during the Depression. Some of the major industries were the Duncan Foundry, the Alton Box Board Company, Owens Illinois Glass Co., Alton Laclede Steel Company, and the Illinois Terminal Railroad company. The latter was where my father worked as a locomotive engineer. The river provided work for men on barges as they moved coal, oil and other supplies up and down these waters. Nearby were other communities that had both oil companies and an ammunition factory, Western Cartridge Co. Because our city was located about 30 miles west of St. Louis, we had the best of both worlds.

In the late forties and early fifties St. Louis was blessed by the establishment of the McDonnell Aircraft Company which in time employed over 30,000 people. Many of Alton's citizens found employment there. This company later became the Boeing Aircraft Company, and the main headquarters moved to Seattle, Washington. As times have changed, Alton has become more of a commuter town with much industry fading out. At one time the population of Alton was nearing 40.000.

Nowadays, a casino river boat is moored at the riverside in downtown Alton, attracting many tourists. "Old man river" is still rolling along, and if you ever lived most of your life on the banks of this river, you miss it terribly should you move elsewhere. I now live on the banks of the Arkansas River in Tulsa, Oklahoma area. Although Tulsa is a beautiful city, her river falls short of the mighty Alton waters. Few if any other rivers can take her place!

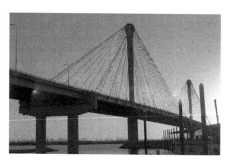

Clark Bridge Alton IL Photo by Illinois2011 Wikimedia Commons

Part III Institutional Life – The Way It Was

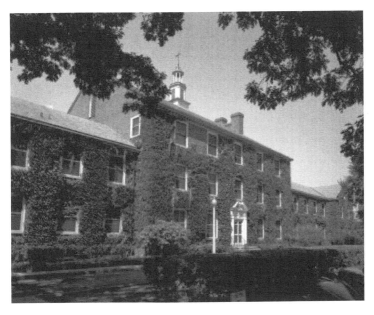

Alton Memorial Hospital 1940s Photo from BJC Healthcare Pinterest page
Historic photos

THE HOSPITALS

The institutions of this day all operated similarly. Management style was the same and male leadership dominated most institutions. Leadership was almost deified. Institutions expected unquestioning loyalty, and this was particularly true in hospitals, churches, schools, and politics. Institutions were heavy on rules and regulations coinciding with a paternalistic milieu of the day. Were these rules all reasonable and necessary? Probably not, but it was still a day when challenging those in charge was just not readily done. Sometimes it appears we have gone overboard in the other direction. We have to have some system clarifying lines of authority for productivity and progress to be made.

The lay clients left patient care decisions up to the physician, who to them represented an authority figure. The doctor was highly respected. At this time there was no such thing as a Patient Bill of Rights. We also had little or no quality control mechanisms or other means for review of methods used in evaluating care of patients.

The most commonly seen medical patients in the smaller hospitals were those with diabetes, heart problems, stomach ulcers, colitis, cirrhosis of the liver, pneumonia, urinary tract infections, and lung problems such as COPD or bronchiectasis. Coronary heart patients were bedridden for seven days or more. Heart surgeries done today were not on the horizon and many coronary patients died who would survive today. No stents or artery bypasses were done. Cancer patients did not, of course, have the advanced therapies now used. The common surgical patients seen were hernia repairs, appendectomies, D&Cs (dilation and curettage of the uterus), hysterectomies, hernia repair, tonsillectomies, circumcisions, eye surgery for cataracts, prostatectomies (transurethral prostatectomy or a supra-pubic prostatectomy), repair of fractured hips or other broken bones, cystoscopies, gallbladder removal, the suturing of cuts, and amputations. Mastectomy surgery was very new and hysterectomies seemed to be one of the main surgical procedures for women.

There seemed to be tendency for some women my mother's age (those born from 1900 to 1925) to frequent doctors' offices and take a lot of medicine. If they did not get what they wanted, they went from doctor to doctor. In no way is my study scientific in nature, but it is interesting to ponder the causes and effects in this behavior. A friend of mine, a psychologist, agreed that these women had been caught in a changing society without the education, skills and self-esteem necessary for them to fit in or feel comfortable or of value. She further referred to this phenomenon as the "Lost Generation of Women". Medically they were called hypochondriacs.

Could this phenomenon not be traced to some unmet needs or damaged self-perception of their earlier

31

formative years and the status of women during those
years? Women were not permitted to vote until 1918;
they were discouraged from getting an education
beyond 8th grade; blamed for bringing sin into the
world; criticized if they found work outside of the
home; were not seen as leaders; and not treated equally
in many areas of society. These women turned to
unhealthy coping strategies and became a burden to
their families and an enigma for doctors who had not a
clue about how to understand these women, let alone
how to treat them.

Freud himself held a disparaging view of women and
this was likely passed on to physicians in his writings
and teachings. Women were viewed as "trouble". In
some of his writings, in addition to his Oedipus
Complex theory, he remarked that in all his thirty years
of research he never could figure out what woman
wanted. Well, *duh!* What else is new?

Personally, I think these women who had little
opportunity to prepare for a changing world wanted to
feel good about themselves and know they had value.
Was this asking too much?

How extreme were the attitudes about women? Well
check out the 1904 article in the *American Medical Journal
of Medicine* that declared it was unhealthy for women to
tax their brain with learning and implied that genital
anomalies were now on the rise due to this mental
overtaxing. This resulted, the article implied, in an
increase in infertility. Really! Do you not understand,

now, why women living in this era might have had "problems"?

Knowing some of this history should make us women appreciate the progress made in women's issues since those days. You do not have to agree with everything the women's' movement has or still is advocating but, as usual, to make society change requires, at times, radical means. Too bad humans cannot make needed changes without extreme pressure. I am not an extreme feminist nor do I hate men or doctors, but I can understand how I would have felt living in the climate my mother had to endure. But in time even such activist groups can overextend their power, become too political, create their own biases, and express animosity toward those who differ with their views, This results in society facing a whole set of new problems.

Gender discrimination did not extend only to women. Men were not encouraged to enter nursing, and in some cases were denied entrance into nursing schools. Women had to fight to enter into law, and medicine. The number of men and non-Caucasians admitted into nursing programs was minimal. Nursing students had to stand in the presence of a doctor. I kid you not! Now I have to admit nurses looked up to the doctors and so did society. They put them on a pedestal and, of course, the male physicians loved it. If you are worshiped as a king, you are not likely to turn that status down. We cannot blame doctors today for those beliefs and behaviors of the past.

Physicians have come a long way since then as you will find many of them employ nurses, male and female, who are clinical specialists to assist them, and have found them to be a tremendous asset to their practice. I was attended by one recently in my son-in-law's practice and I told my daughter "Hiring her was the smartest thing he ever did." Well, actually, it was the second smartest thing. Marrying my daughter was the first, along with getting me as a mother in law!

Racial discrimination in the health care system came as a shock to me as a young student nurse. This realization occurred when I first learned that white and black patients were segregated in most hospitals. This should never have occurred but thankfully this policy was beginning to change across the nation. Admission of non-white applicants into previously Caucasian-only nursing programs also became a reality for minorities.

OUR CHURCHES

I have tremendous respect for our religious institutions, although, because they are made up of humans, they are not now, nor were they ever, perfect. A variety of churches of various denominations could be found in our community. Each, of course, thought they were the most pure in doctrine. I used to think, "Gee, if we are the only ones going to heaven in this town, this city is in bad shape." But God gave me many opportunities to associate with many Christians of various churches and I concluded very quickly that the main doctrine that counts is the one about Christ being our Savior.

This complete trust in authority carried over to the parishioner's attitude towards the clergy and church leaders, who, yes, were mostly male. After all, these men were expected to be more educated and trustworthy and more knowledgeable about the scriptures. Most churches expected loyalty to the denomination, as well, and interfaith mixing or socializing was not strongly encouraged.

There was a movement in our country at that time espousing the idea that "God is dead". Battles took place between liberals and conservatives over doctrine and the inspiration of the Bible. People had great fear of the growth of communism. Billy Graham was a young evangelist who had not yet achieved the height of his fame. Pope Pius XII was at the Vatican.

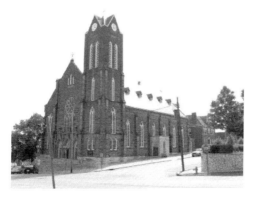

St. Mary's Catholic Church of Alton. Photo by Kim Foster on City Data

Yes, religious prejudice was common and it went in all directions. My Catholic cousins and I felt a distance between us until we became adults, when we became close. Catholics were not to attend a non-Catholic church and many Protestants would not attend a Catholic church.

By going to school with kids from other faiths, we found out that most of us worshiped the same Savior who died on the cross for our sins. One classmate asked me, "Do you think God will hear the prayer of a Baptist for a Catholic?" Her mother was sick and she wanted prayer for her. Well, since neither one of us knew the answer to her question for sure, and had little contact with people of other faiths, we decided to give it a try, anyway. We felt that it would be okay. Most of our churches were racially segregated then, but at least apologies have been made. That situation has greatly improved and many interracial congregations now exist.

Personal living guidelines were prescribed and some were more man-made than biblically mandated. It was not appropriate for women to wear pants and never in church. Long hair for boys and men was definitely out. Drinking any alcoholic beverages, movie attendance, dancing, smoking, card playing, and such, were sins according to many churches. A chain of command interpretation of the headship role for men in the family was generally the rule, not the exception. Some churches today still hold to this order of family relations with men having the leadership position. Well, women may not have been officially deaconesses in their churches, but from my observations growing up, they had a way of being heard. Oh, yes, you women know what I mean. Today, more denominations approve of women ministers and deaconesses and allow women to have a greater role in the decision-making process. I am just stating how things were then and are now.

Even styles of worship change and are often a result of generational preferences in worship and music. My church sang the traditional hymns and gospel songs and had a more non-liturgical worship service while others had a semi-to fully liturgical worship order. Today we find the very contemporary music and worship style versus the traditional services. The contemporary generation seems to be setting the style.

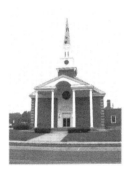

Calvary Baptist Church, Alton, IL, from the church website

In spite of what some may view as hangups and even inequities, the church did play a significant positive role in emphasizing the Christian life; teachings and examples of Christ, and the Judeo-Christian standards for morality and ethical values. It taught the love of God, country, and others. It provided a sense of acceptance and an extended family support system.

Many young nursing students who were raised in such
an atmosphere developed a strong altruistic desire to
serve others, such as in nursing, while other young
women went into teaching or even missionary service.
What would the world be like without Lottie Moon,
Mother Teresa, Florence Nightingale, and Clara Barton!

It is not the in-vogue thing today to say I feel a "calling"
to go into nursing. Is it so wrong to feel that way? I, as a
Christian, make no apology for my faith in Christ. There
is no better profession than nursing or medicine for one
to sense the presence of God and experience miracles
of healing that have no human explanation. I have seen
the results of prayer in my life and work and in the lives
of my patients and students that could have only come
from a higher power.

I do not, nor have I ever, pushed my religion off onto
others in my line of teaching or nursing. I chose to let
my life demonstrate a difference by sharing my love,
compassion and also my faith and prayers, as
appropriate. I presently serve as a caring Stephen
minister in my church and continue to respond to those
who are hurting or need help.

I taught back in the late 60's when young people were
protesting and using hallucinogenic drugs like LSD.
One young man came into my office to ask if he could
enter my nursing program. I had filled up the class and
told him I would review his situation and get back with
him. When he came back, I told him I was going to let
him enroll into the program. He looked at me and said,
"Gee, I guess prayer does work." He had told me about

his drug involvement. After this young man graduated, one day he was working in a hospital about 35 miles away. I was at my desk when the phone rang. A male voice started quoting me scripture and I thought it was a *nut* but then he called me by name and said that he had been walking down the hall and the Lord told him to "call Mrs. Wilson as she was discouraged", which was true. The hair stood up on my arms as this was a God thing! He thanked me for giving him the Word, referring to the Gideon nurses' white Testament that was offered at pinning ceremonies. No one was required to take the Testaments. It was voluntary.

No, Mark did not actually hear an audible voice. He responded to that small nudge from the Holy Spirit to make that call. Some will call this intuition. That is their choice. Mark turned out to be one of my many fine graduates. Was this just a coincidence that our paths had crossed? I think not! I could cite many other incidences similar to this one in the course of my long life. I highly recommend the Christian life. It certainly has worked for me.

I want to encourage you who are in nursing or maybe still a nursing student to wear your faith proudly, but do it with love and tolerance for those who are anti-religious or neutral. You can do more by living out Christ-like behaviors than by being judgmental. Your life is an instrument that Christ uses to bring physical, emotional, and/or spiritual healing to others. Your faith is part of who you are and cannot be separated from you.

OUR *SCHOOLS*

I do not remember having racial disturbances in the school system during my time but I was aware of racial prejudice as this was before the Civil Rights Movement. But of course the number of non-Caucasians who attended our school was small. During my school days, from my standpoint, I sensed that a distinction, if and when made, was based more on economic status than on racial basis.

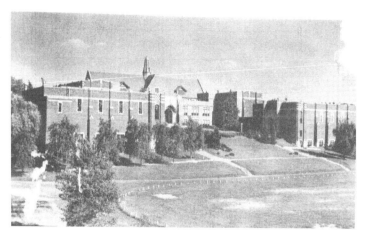

Alton High School, photo from the author's personal collection

Our school system at that time, as memory serves me, rated very highly academically. A beautiful older high school sat below the new East Junior High School on College Avenue. We always had an outstanding high school band. Football was, of course, a given, and the annual contest between Western Military Academy and Alton High was a must to attend on Thanksgiving Day, even though the weather many times was so cold your cheeks would become numb. But who cared! This was life at its best, especially if Alton High won the game.

Our community also had a Catholic High School, Marquette High School. We also had a small college, Shurtleff College, which I attended and obtained my Bachelor of Science degree following my nursing training. It was an American Baptist College but is now a branch of Southern Illinois University. Western Military Academy is now a private Christian School operated by the Faith Baptist Church in Godfrey, Ill. North of Alton was a small community of Godfrey, Illinois and it had a girl's private college, called Monticello College, which became Lewis and Clark Community College. With St. Louis being so near, two major universities were accessible if students wanted to attend. These schools were St. Louis University and Washington University. The latter one I attended to obtain my Masters in Nursing. Southern Illinois University was built in Edwardsville, Illinois which is about 30 mile east of Alton and its other campus exist in Carbondale, Ill.

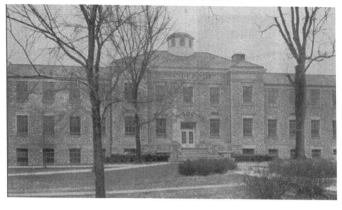

Shurtleff College Historical Archive Photo

ECONOMIC PICTURE

The economic portrait of this community resulted mainly from industry and the union influence. Salaries were slowly improving but families still struggled. During the Depression men were making 25 to 27 cents an hour which was the starting point from which salaries rose after the Depression. We students came from low to high-medium income families with the majority being between the upper low to the median range. We lived rather frugally but hoped for a better future. We could sense it and then we began to realize it.

As a side note, Depression children bore the marks of the Depression years and took on some of their parents traits as stocking up on food items. My mother and aunts stored cans of Spry (like Crisco) pounds of sugar, bars of soap, etc. As adults they were cautious in their spending even when finances were so much improved. Even now I have several boxes of toothpaste and soap in my bathroom. My generation seemed to be conservative in spending even though things were much better for our generation economically.

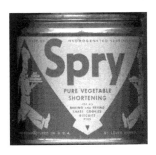

Can of Spry. Photo from timepassagesnostalgia.com

Work opportunities made it possible to find some kind of employment. The bread lines no longer existed, and life was looking up in our country. Industry at midcentury was growing in St. Louis area and surrounding communities. A new McDonnell Aircraft company began to provide many good jobs for the next 50 years. My husband worked there for 42 years. The company eventually became Boeing Airlines with its headquarters in Seattle, Washington.

We nursing students were given a stipend at the insistence of the Methodist Church, and although it was not a lot, it was a godsend to us students.

We received $5 a month the first year; $10 a month the second year; and $15 a month the third year. It was amazing what we could do with that amount of money.

Not all of the classes received this stipend. In fact, our class may have been the only class. My starting salary in 1950 was $200 per month. Wow! But I was able to buy a new Studebaker.

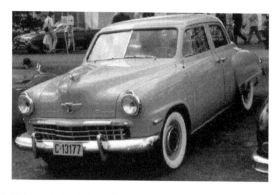

Approx. 1949 Studebaker Photo Lars-Göran Lindgren Wikimedia Commons

SOCIAL LIFE

Not many families dined out or went to many outside entertainment places. Television was not on the radar for most families as yet. Picnicking in the community park, participating in community centers, swimming in public pools, and attending school and church social functions provided social outlets for the families. For those who could afford it, additional educational, recreational, dining, and cultural resources could be found just across the river in St. Louis, Missouri. The home, church, or school made up the social hubs for most families.

The big chain, name restaurants we have today were not available back then. Drive-in eating places had not appeared on the scene. Yes, we had no McDonalds. Because St. Louis was so close, we were able to attend the St. Louis Cardinal games if the family budget would allow. A streetcar ran between Alton and St. Louis which made it possible for those who had no car to travel to St. Louis. The St. Louis Zoo and the art museum were favorite spots for a visit.

And so you have a flavor of our community which influenced our upbringing. I have tried to be honest and point out the good and the weaknesses that I observed. Every generation has it warts. Yours will have some also. Prejudices occur when people have had little contact with other races or religions, or lack of education opportunities. Yes, society is slow to change but in time it does occur. Never think that your society has arrived at perfection.

No, ours was not a perfect world. But it was the world we were given. Our world gave us a chance to learn from the past and change what we could for the present and hopefully for the future, especially, in alleviating the pain of the human condition. Nursing was our way. We got our start in the professional world and built upon it by additional experiences and educational opportunities. These opportunities prepared us to make needed changes in nursing care and nursing education for future students and patients. Our community and the hospital they built gave us this chance!

We Diploma students were oblivious to the conflict that existed between hospitals, medicine, and nursing. I do know this generation of young women met the challenge and the proof is in the lasting endurance and contribution of these caring and capable Registered Nurses these past sixty years. May the new nurse be as blessed.

So with this background, I now am ready to allow you to travel with me along this three-year journey in the life of a Diploma student nurse. I assure you it will not be dull. You will gain an appreciation for those who cared for the sick; facing situations not seen today; under working conditions not allowed today; and who cared enough to accept these challenges without whining or protesting, as some might do today. No one can describe it but one who lived it. And so now, I will accompany you to a time of unique conditions and special people. Just open the door and enter into the halls that will lead to a life-changing experience.

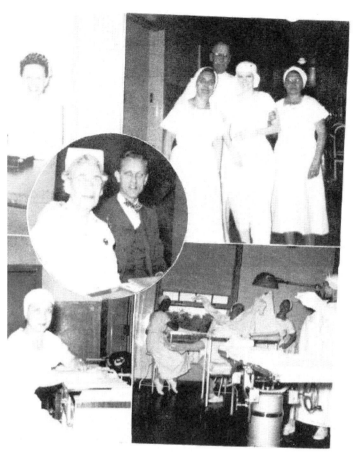

School Life – Yearbook Page

Part IV A Three-Year, Life-Changing Journey

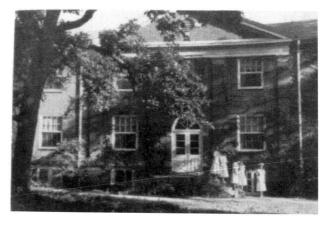

Mary Hall Alton Hospital Nursing School. From Author's Yearbook

NURSING: AN ESSENCE OF GRACE

Put on your nursing cap, say a prayer, and come with me through the halls of time and up and down hospital corridors. Imagine you are living through the experiences that we will recall. Pass beyond the hospital doors into a world all its own. You will become part of human drama that intertwines lives with a whole gamut

48

of intense emotions played out on a stage we know as a patient unit. Here decisions and actions must be made quickly and accurately, under stressful conditions, knowing that what you do may make a difference between life and death.

The word *compassion* takes on a unique meaning for those in the health field. Max Lucado, a minister and author expresses it this way: "Compassion comes from a Greek word *splanchnology* meaning 'hurt in the gut'." A compassionate nurse feels the patient's pain; his fears; his anxiety; and his loneliness deep in the gut, so to speak. True compassion, then, becomes grace in action. The nurse learns that through pain character becomes weaker or stronger, bitter or better, and through suffering personal growth is hindered or enhanced. Through the sharing of tender loving care to another human being one can give hope and comfort for the sufferer.

And so there comes to be a co-mingling of feelings between the patient and the nurse; one human heart is getting to know another human heart as they pulsate together.

Our patients had rather long hospital stays, so the nurse was able to know her patient. Often a surgical patient was in bed for 7 days and, of course, medicine learned this practice was not wise and predisposed the patient to blood clots. But medicine has never been an absolute science. Mistakes were and are made but learning ensues. Jokingly you hear folk saying "that is why they call it medical *practice*!"

The patient has a goal of getting well and the nurse assists in achieving that goal. The patient hurts and the nurse attempts to ease that pain. The nurse's hand is sensitive to the coolness or warmth. She notes the color of the patient's skin. She reads the eyes to detect fear or detects the significance of a change of the size of the pupil, or sees a tear that may be falling on the cheek. The nurse watches the hands to see if they are steady or trembling; she listens to the breathing to hear any panting or breathlessness; and her sense of smell picks up any odor that may help in a diagnosis or change a course of treatment. All the nurse's senses are activated.

Tenderly and astutely the nurse cares for the patient, observing, listening, and interpreting all the time. The nurse becomes attuned to sensing changes unobservable to others. She knows intuitively at times, that something is wrong. She listens to her heart when it says "go back and check one more time." It pays off when a patient has fallen out of bed. The nurse finds much joy when the patient recovers but feels great loss and even failure when the patient loses the battle.

The nurse and the doctor are caught in this emotional drama and between those two and the patient, the souls of three people form a triangle and a bond. The patient is the focus. The nurse and the doctor become a team. The nurse becomes the eyes and ears of the doctor. He prescribes a plan of medical treatment and the nurse carries out his instructions, although really a healing partnership exists, and the doctor who listens to the nurse's suggestions is wise. Both know a life is in their hands. The nurse has to remember the doctor takes an oath to save lives, not lose lives. And so death is hard for the doctor to accept. The nurse is more likely to be present when death does occur. Dealing with the grief of the family also becomes the nurse's charge.

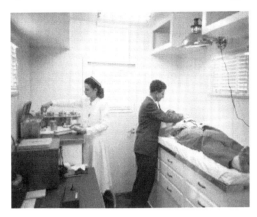

Doctor and nurse in examining room HRC photograph collection pre 1950s.

The nurse has great respect for a doctor who is good at what he/she does. A doctor knows the nurse he is most likely to trust. Her knowledge of specific diseases, signs, and symptoms, enables her to be astute, assessing critical changes taking place with the patient and discerning when to consult with the physician.

The nurse and the patient's family become involved. Attending to their needs is helpful and comforting to the patient. Communication skills are essential for the nurse and can go a long way in allaying fears of the family and comforting them.

Such is the environment within these halls. A plethora of emotional situations, ranging from anxiety, depression, mourning, fear, anger, hopelessness; but then joy at sometimes miraculous, unexplainable recoveries. Nursing is an art requiring care that demonstrates knowledge, compassion, technical proficiency, communication skills, observational acuity, emotional maturity, and discernment. It was a tall order for one who dared to cross the threshold to step beyond these open doors, not knowing her life would change forever.

STEPPING BEYOND THE OPEN DOORS

It was September, 1947, and I, a very frightened 17-year-old, found myself looking at beautiful, ornate white doors and fearfully grabbing hold of the knob. I walked into the charming lobby of Alton Memorial Hospital. I turned to watch my father drive away and felt a sinking feeling in the pit of my stomach. My heart thumped so loud I feared others could hear. I was leaving my sheltered environment and family to become part of a new family and assume a new life.

Other young women sat in the lobby looking just as frightened as I felt. I sat down by the person who was going to become my roommate, Grace German, although neither of us knew that we would live together literally for the next three years. Grace was a quiet, reserved individual like me, so we made a compatible combination.

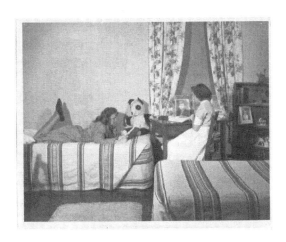

Dorm room BJC Healthcare pinterest page historic Alton Hospital photos

I did not realize where this new life would take me nor could I ever have imagined this was a start of what became a very productive and rewarding career, taking me from bedside nursing to teaching, directing and developing nursing programs, to vice president of patient care. Had I had any idea, my timidity would have caused me to run, for my self-esteem was not very high. So I am grateful for the start I received that September day in 1947.

An elderly nurse came into the lobby and asked that we all follow her down to the chapel where we would receive our orientation. This nurse was the director of the Nursing School and of the Hospital, but was leaving this position in a short time. Her name was Ms. Hortense Stafford and I would guess her age to be nearing or in her early 70s. After leaving her position as Director she did private duty nursing.

She lived near my home and many a time people would drive up Main Street hill headed for Upper Alton and, lo and behold, they would see this elderly lady back her car out into the street from her garage, stop and park it, get out, go back, shut her garage door, then return to her car and only then move it out of the way of oncoming traffic. You see, life was taken at a more causal pace back then. What was the big rush? Road rage! Unknown to us.

A young woman, age 29, replaced Ms. Stafford in 1948, Ms. Virginia Cramblet, who was the Director of Nursing and Educational Director for the next twenty-plus years. She saw nursing education change and the handwriting on the wall for Diploma programs. Both schools of nursing in Alton closed and the nursing programs came under the auspices of Lewis and Clark Community College in Godfrey, Illinois, (formerly Monticello College) in 1971. Alton Memorial had graduated 417 female and 9 male students and had served this community well. The last class graduated in 1973.

As fate would have it, I, had the privilege of directing this new program and graduating eight classes of Associate Degree nurses. Ms. Cramblet had a major role in my becoming the one to take over the reins of this new program after it had gotten into serious difficulty the first year. I was at that moment Director of Nursing at St. Mary's Hospital in East St. Louis, Illinois. I was approached by the college administration to assume the duties of re-directing its development.

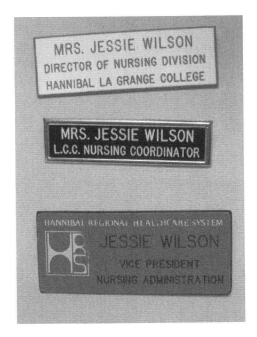

Identification tags for some of the nursing positions held by the author

It became not only an accredited program by State of Illinois but was granted accreditation by the National League of Nursing. The percentage of state board successes was 98 %. The first class graduated in the spring of 1973. I remained the director of this program until fall of 1981 and left to develop a new Associate Degree and Bachelor Degree completion nursing programs at Hannibal LaGrange College, in Hannibal, Missouri, now Hannibal-LaGrange University.

There are many of my students, now, graduates who are practicing nursing somewhere today, whose lives this Diploma nurse touched. It is thrilling to know that *touch* will be passed on through these former students. I still hear from some of them who write and express appreciation for being under my tutelage. They, however, gave much more to enrich my life.

Now, let's return to 1947, as I strayed a little bit. Ms. Stafford informed us of our dorm room number and who our roommate would be, and then came the rules. Oh yes, this was the day of rules and regulations. Some seemed excessive but our parents did not think so. Here are just some of them:

1. No smoking or drinking on the grounds

2. No shorts or pants could be worn

3. No marriage while in school

4. Chapel attendance each morning was mandatory

5. No personal involvement with a physician

6. Signing in and out when leaving the dorm was required.

7. Curfew on weekends was enforced

8. Hem of student uniform was to be no shorter than 13 inches above the ground

9. Lights out at 10 p.m.

10. House mother to check rooms every night after lights out.

Note: Any infraction of rules would result in disciplinary action varying from dismissal to being confined to the grounds for period of time which was called "being campused".

Such was our life when living on campus and everyone had to live on the grounds.

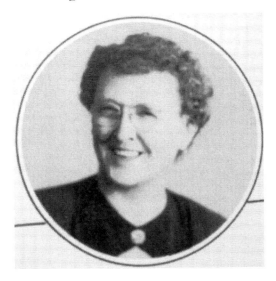

Mrs. Edna Loomis. Picture from the school yearbook.

The school had two new nursing dormitories which would become our home away from home for the next three years. The one was called Mary Hall and the other Martha Hall. The accommodations were very homey, attractive, and well furnished. Each home had a housemother who lived in the dorm. A Mrs. Mary White was over Martha Hall and a Mrs. Edna Loomis was over Mary Hall, two very sweet, older, gracious Christian women. They became our surrogate mothers and let us cry on their shoulders in times of discouragements, while always urging us onward.

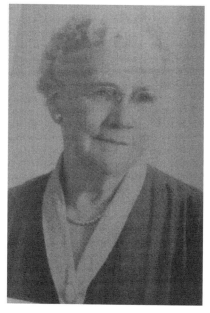

Mary White. Yearbook Photo

Now, I would not want you to believe that we students back then did not ever break the rules. You know rules are made to be broken, right? Students are very imaginative in discovering ways to get around rules that don't quite make sense to them. For example, the dorm always had a first floor with windows that could be climbed in and out of with the help of our classmates. Our mothers never raised any dummies, so wearing shorts under our skirts until we got off campus was pretty easy to do. Marriages did occur but could not be made public as dismissal would result.

We often waited until the dorm mother had made her bed checks and then got into our closets to study. We just had to make sure the light did not shine under the door. Just wanted you to know we were normal young people. Years later, while I was teaching at St. Joseph Hospital School of Nursing, a group of students escaped through the windows one night and they were caught and were in deep trouble with the good Sister. We faculty had to act chagrined, as well, but they were a good bunch of kids, and underneath we were smiling. I know the AMH students were known to do the same at times. But *never* yours truly!

After hearing the rules spelled out to us, we were measured for our student uniform, which was a blue-checked dress with white starched cuffs and collar. After our *probie* (probation) time a white bib and a starched apronlike skirt were added over the dress. You can imagine we got a little warm in the summer months The nursing cap could not be worn until we had gone through the first 6 months of probation. This is why we were called *probies*. White oxford shoes and white hose, a watch with a second hand, a pen, and a pair of bandage scissors completed the dress requirement.

Next, we received our textbooks and class schedule. We would not be going to the hospital for four months. Classes that we would be taking the first semester included the following: Anatomy and Physiology, Nursing Arts, Chemistry, Pharmacology I, Nursing History, and Microbiology. The really fun class was Nursing Arts which took place in our hospital lab room with hospital beds and adult patient dolls, named Mr. and Mrs. Chase. Our nursing instructors would show us how to do various nursing procedures and observe our practice on these dolls. These dolls were nothing compared to what the today's students have to practice on. Wow! I think they are so programmed they can tell the students what to do. Almost!

Our upper-class students would often play a trick on us by removing the adult dolls and lying in the beds, and when we would come into the class lab, they would rise up and scare us. They also would play other little jokes on us when we finally got into the hospital. For example, knowing we had very little knowledge of anatomy as yet, one would say, "Hey, Glover (my maiden name) go up to Central supply and bring me down a package of Fallopian tubes." Thinking these were some rubber tubing, like catheters, or something like that I, of course, went, only to be told that I had been *had!*

I am not sure my mother knew she had Fallopian tubes, either. In fact, talking about body parts was not a likely discussion. By the time our mothers got around to telling us about the joy of the monthly cycle, we of course were already well-educated on that subject. Our grandmothers used another expression for the whole experience. My aunt asked me one time when I was about 12, "Has your granny come yet?" Trying not to laugh, I looked at her and seriously replied, "No, she does not know I am in town." She looked at another aunt and they rolled their eyes at one another, thinking, "My, word, is this kid dumb or what?" Now, I do not know how that expression ever was dreamed up when talking about the onset of womanhood.

In Pharmacology I, we learned how to calculate drug problems. As I mentioned earlier, we did not have pre-packaged medications or even calculators. We had to know how to use algebraic equations for our drug problems. We would have to take the quantity we had on hand and determine how much of it to use or not use when the dosage ordered by the doctor varied. The doctor might have ordered a solution of 30% and we might have had a solution of 50% so we had to know how to add the right amount of diluent to get the strength ordered. We had no machines to regulate the dripping of I.V. drops per minute. So again we had to calculate how many drips per minute to regulate the number of c.c.s to be given in the amount of time ordered by the doctor. It was necessary to know the metric system of meters, liters, and kilograms as well as apothecary systems of grains, grams, etc.

Learning to give injections was done by practicing on oranges. A brave instructor might occasionally offer to be a guinea pig. We learned how to start an intravenous injections and this, of course, was more difficult and required a good sense of touch to find a good vein. Veins can fool you. It may look like a good one but often it is what we called the rolling, rubbery kind and was difficult to stick. Keep in mind we did not have disposable, pre-packaged, sterile equipment. The tubing was thick rubber and everything had to be packaged, sterilized, cleansed, and re-sterilized in autoclaves found in Central Supply.

Administering narcotics was a serious business and we had to retrieve them out of a locked cabinet, sign out for them, and put down how many tablets or vials were left. At the end of each shift a nurse was responsible to check to see if the count was right and no narcotic missing. It was true back then, as it is now, that occasionally a nurse would manage to take narcotics and falsely report the count. It is much harder now to do this but when it occurs it is a sad thing. The person will get caught, resulting in the suspension or loss of his or her licenses to practice nursing.

And so, having learned many nursing procedures used in patient care, the day arrived when we were able to start our clinical practice for real. The moment of truth had come and our schedule for each day became as follows: clinical practice 7:00 a.m. to 11 a.m.; class 12-3 p.m.; clinical practice 3-7 p.m.; study time 7-9 p.m.; lights out at 10:00 p.m. Now, this became our normal day during our first year.

Remember, however, that it took many years later before the schedule of the medical interns were found to be even more overwhelming, even to the point of being dangerous. I think a concern, and rightly so, of the nursing leaders, was that often with nursing instructors spread too thin, the nursing staff often could be too busy to take responsibility for the student. The student would be on her own, making decisions that affected the patients but really needed a Registered Nurses' knowledge and experience. I ask though, do the present day students have a one-on-one instructor/ mentor with them at all times? I doubt it?

It did help that any new procedure or treatment we learned under the supervision of an instructor had to be done correctly at least three times. We never graduated without having executed the required procedures and, if for some reason if we made three errors, we were in danger of being removed from the program. We also realized the importance of seeking help in any situation where we felt inadequate. The number three has some significance, as things seemed to happen in threes. Three babies would be born in one night, or three deaths would occur in one day, etc. Also, the changing of the moon had some effect on events, and I bet most of today's nurses would agree.

THE PROBIE MEETS THE PATIENT

Entering the patient units or wards as some were called was a very serious but exciting time. We were welcomed by the nursing staff which consisted of head nurses, staff registered nurses, nurse aids, male orderlies, and then the nursing students. Most were gracious to us and did all they could do to help us and teach us. Since our two clinical nursing instructors could not oversee all of us probies at one time, the other members of the staff pitched in. I have to admit, the graduate nurses were

most helpful, and they actually were our mentors. We
shadowed them but never knew that was the term.

It was these Diploma Registered Nurses who taught us
how to perfect our skills. Most of them were new
graduates themselves, having studied in the early-or-
mid-1940s. Some had been in the cadet nursing
programs during world War II. Each student was
assigned one of these R.Ns as our big sister.

The orderlies in our hospital were men who had been
medics in World War II and, were two brothers, Bob
and Cliff Strange. The doctors utilized these men to
assist with the post-op prostate surgery patients and
orthopedic patients. I think they did more than the
usual orderly was supposed to do. They were good and
no one questioned that fact. They were extremely skilled
in starting I.V.s (intravenous injections). They were very
helpful to the students, even if they did play jokes on
them once in a while.

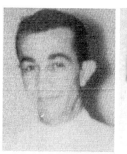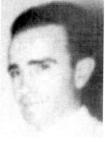

Strange Brothers, Orderlies at the school, from the Nursing Yearbook

One time, as the story goes, some new students were
asked to take a corpse down to the morgue. The

students were unaware that one of the orderlies lay on the stretcher covered up with a sheet. He waited until they were on the elevator and then he rose up. Of course, you can imagine the shock. Also, in our classroom lab hung a skeleton. One day it had a bikini on, with a bra that was greatly oversized and stuffed. On this day, a dignified clergyman was on campus touring. This made the trick even more hilarious. In a small hospital, the personnel spent so much time together that they became family. Creating humor did help to lessen the stress.

There were certain head nurses whom we liked better than others. Most were kind but firm. A dear older nurse, Mrs. Holt, was a hard worker and she could go, or more like it, run, up and down those halls faster than any of us youngsters. Sometimes she would go ahead and do the task at hand rather than take the time to explain it to us. We admired her, though, and we would think, "Gee I want to be just like her."

The Registered Nurses who worked with us have to be given much credit for being good role models. Certainly I have never experienced in my forty year nursing career such gentle, caring, and competent individuals. We students idolized them and dreamed of being that kind of nurse. They were confident and, yes, gracious ladies who inspired, encouraged, and instructed us in the art of nursing. The majority of them were, as I stated earlier, AMH graduates, or nurses who had returned from serving in one of the Women's Military Corps, or had trained in the Cadet Nursing program.

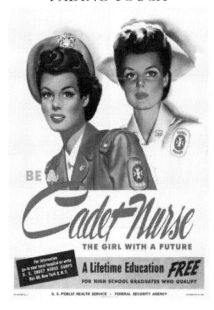

US Government Printing Office; Pritzker Military Library, Chicago, IL

They took us aside when they observed that we were falling apart in crisis situations. These could range from a patient who was hemorrhaging to one who was dying. They soothed our hurt feelings if a physician vented his wrath on us, as some would occasionally do. Perhaps we even deserved it. They shared little tricks of the trade they had learned that we did not read about in textbooks. It was Ms. Crabtree, Ms. Shewmaker, Mrs. Perrin, Mrs. Bennett, and many others who inspired and invested, in essence, part of themselves in us, for our learning and edification.

As probie students we were assigned patients to bathe, give back rubs, change their bed sheets, assist in feeding, run errands for the staff, etc. As we learned new basic techniques in the nursing lab then we would begin to perform these procedures on our patients. Many of these tasks today have been taken over by nursing assistants.

The medical staff was mostly kind to us students, although, you always have those who were arrogant and intimidating to students and even staff nurses. Two older doctors, Dr. Williamson and Dr. Pfiffenberger, would come into the unit wearing hats and each would tip his hat to the nurses. I never heard either one raise his voice to the nurse. But this new younger doctor was a new breed!

Some felt like they could do anything and get away with it and you know what? They probably were right! Others, you were afraid to call in the middle of the night and wake them from their sleep. You would hear expletives that you had never heard. Others would be grateful you called, especially if the patient was in distress. The latter were those doctors whom we respected, and one cannot let a few spoil everyone in a group. As a whole, our groups of doctors at that time were considered good at what they did.

One of the most stressing skills for us early on was making the bed with the patient in it. Not only did we have to deal with the patient, rolling him over, back, and forth as we changed sides, but the draw sheet had to be just so. The draw sheet was a about four-feet wide. It went crosswise over the bottom sheet in the middle of the bed and tucked in on each side. It had to be so tight that one could toss a coin on it and it would bounce up in the air. Both bed sheets were flat sheets and the

corners had to be mitered smoothly. The tightness of
the draw sheet practice is traced back to the way military
personnel had to make up their cots. Why the carryover
into nursing, I cannot tell you, except that many of our
graduates had been in the service during World War II,
and I presume they brought this practice with them.

I do know that wrinkles can be a factor in the
development of bed sores. We students knew our
bedmaking would be checked out by our instructors, so
we would make them very tight and tell the patients,
who would be lying with toes straight up, "Please don't
move until our instructor comes in and makes her
evaluation." Have you ever lain in bed with a tight sheet
pressing on your toes and felt comfortable?

While learning about skills in Nursing Arts class, our
other classes taught us about the body structures and
how our organs functioned. I am not sure why it was
important to memorize the origin and insertions of all
the muscles. We learned each of the cranial nerves by
the following ditty: *On Old Olympus Towering Top, a Fin
and German Viewed some Hops* (dances). The first letter of
each word of this rhyme stood for these cranial nerves:
Olfactory, Optic, Oculomotor, Trochlear, Trigeminal,
Abducens, Facial, Auditory, Glossopharyngeal, Vagus,
Spinal Accessory, and Hypoglossal.

Chemistry was a drag, but I still remember the symbol
NACL stands for sodium chloride or salt. For chemistry
we met with the students from St. Joseph Hospital and
a nun taught us. I was intrigued by the sister's habit,
especially the large, starched head-covering which is

called the cornette or, in some cases, a veil. I was more interested in knowing if the nuns had to cut their hair than in concentrating on Chemistry. Even when God placed this Baptist as Director of a Catholic hospital many moons later, I did not have the courage to ask that question. I do know that my two-year-old daughter ran and hid behind our couch when one of these good sisters came to visit me years later. It was embarrassing. Their head coverings truly were huge, and they looked like the sisters in the *Flying Nun* TV series.

In Pharmacology II we would study all about the drugs we would be administering. The day I learned one should count the pulse before giving Digoxin and if the count was below 60 you were to withhold the drug, I nearly had a heart attack. I had given it that morning and had not counted the pulse. After class I ran back to see if the patient was okay.

Nursing History gave us an appreciation for Florence Nightingale who is considered the Mother of Nursing. She too nursed in another time and another world and under the worst of worst conditions. She came from a family with means who educated her and was not happy with their daughter's choice of vocation. Life in England at that time was miserable in many ways, but should a young woman have wanted to serve humanity, it was not viewed as appropriate work and was not socially acceptable for moral young women.

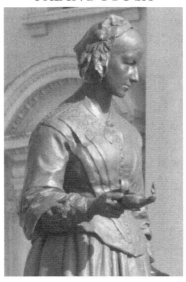

Florence Nightingale by Arthur George Walker. Part of the Crimean War
Memorial, London. Wikimedia Commons

Florence took a nursing team to the Crimean battle
scene and set up a hospital where brave men were
brought when injured. The Bubonic Plague was
prevalent during this time as well. Having no running
water or elevators to carry things up and down the
floors, Florence invented a dumbwaiter to help lighten
the nurses' load. She later developed nursing standards
and even nursing curriculum and standards for training
young women to be nurses. Diploma Nursing programs
originated from her ideas. She is known as the Mother
of Modern-Day Nursing.

Shortly after enrolling in the program I was preparing to
retire one night. I looked out of my window and told
my roommate that I had a peculiar feeling of impending
doom. Early the next morning we students were

suddenly involved in a community disaster. A tornado struck a nearby community and devastated two towns: Bunker Hill, Illinois, and Fosterburg, Illinois. Ten years later another tornado did even more damage. All available hands were called on duty and we found our halls filled with shocked families looking for loved ones who had been injured and brought to the hospital. I found an uncle who had been brought in with an arm gash. He and his wife and two small children had been blown out of their house from their second floor. We students grew up very quickly that day.

Before we knew it, our six-month probationary period was coming to an end. A couple of our classmates had already dropped out, finding the studies beyond their capability, or just feeling that this was not their calling. The drop-out rate was high in nursing schools and some schools often boasted of this, which always seemed strange to me. It was, I assume, a criteria for supposedly a "good school". I really think it showed a deficiency in the selection process. Some say that it proved the overly rigorous schedule of these programs.

We were informed that the capping ceremony would take place, when we would receive our nursing caps. Now I know capping ceremonies are the thing of the past, but for this time period the cap had a lot of significance. It had no sanitary or religious benefit at all to us, but helped identify the nurse for many years.

Nursing history was influenced by Religious Orders and Military life. Some of the rigid rules or disciplinary measures were a carryover, such as the making of cots

used in the military, and the wearing of caps like the
nuns' head coverings. In fact, our cap was sort of like a
miniature copy of the Daughters of Charity head
covering. Each school designed its own caps. Our cap
was made out of a very stiff, starched, square piece of
white material that could be folded into a small peak in
the middle with the wings folded down at the corners.

Of course, there were rules for how it was to be folded
and how tall the peak should be, but after a while we
would make the peak even smaller. We students liked
the peak better that way, and we hoped the director
never noticed.

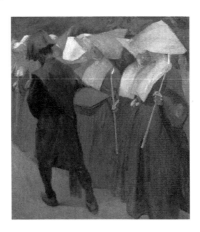

Painting of Daughters of Charity by Karol Tichy from the National Museum
in Warsaw Wikimedia Commons

Now, the real significance of the cap to us was that we
had achieved a milestone. Wearing a cap made us feel
like we were on our way to become a nurse. It made us
feel accepted and gave us an identity. Symbols have
meaning but they come and go as society changes. With
symbols often come rites such as the Florence

Nightingale Capping Ceremony. Because Miss Nightingale had made such an impact on nursing in improving nursing conditions and nursing education, this ceremony for us probies was in honor of "the woman with the lamp" and her unique touch.

The lighting of the Florence Nightingale lamp at the Capping ceremony also endeared nurses to this woman as it was in remembrance of how she was often seen during the Crimean War going from bed to bed at night, checking her soldier patients with her tiny flickering lamp flame. So we each had to carry a Florence Nightingale lamp and one of our instructors dressed as Florence would light our candles. I, as a nursing instructor later on, portrayed Miss Nightingale at several capping ceremonies. I have pictures to prove it. Very serious stuff back then!

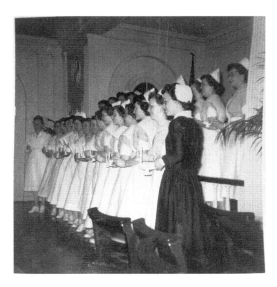

The author portrays Florence Nightingale in a Capping Ceremony – personal photo

In order for us to participate in the ceremony, we had to recite in unison the Florence Nightingale Nursing Pledge from memory. Each of us had to go before the Nursing Director and recite this pledge without making a mistake. This was like judgment day! One of my classmates got so nervous she had to go back in three times before she said the pledge correctly. But Verna was our loveable Lucille Ball. Every class has to have a Lucille.

The pledge goes as follows:

"I solemnly pledge myself in the presence of this assembly to pass my life in purity and practice my profession faithfully. I will abstain from whatever is deleterious and mischievous and will not take or knowingly administer any harmful drug. I will do all in my power to elevate the standard of my profession and will hold in confidence any personal matters committed to my keeping and family affairs coming to my knowledge in the practice of my profession. With loyalty I will endeavor to aid the physician in his work and devote myself to those in my care."

The modern thinking is that the pledge and the cap and capping ceremony are outdated. They are considered by some to be objectionable because the oath implies servitude to the doctor and the ceremony has too much of a spiritual overtone. The white uniform has also taken back seat to a variety of colors and styles.

The ceremony did take on a sort of spiritual overtone, but most of us came from religious backgrounds and it felt right to envision our work as a calling from God and following the teachings of Christ when he stated that "when ye give a drink of water unto the least of these (or the *sickest* of these), ye do it unto me." I would like to think that any nurse taking care of me is guided by Judeo-Christian principles, and certainly one that also has that special touch or gift of grace.

With the cap on our heads completing our uniform and a commitment to go forth and further enhance our skills and knowledge with confidence and devotion, we were ready to be promoted to freshman status and assume increased responsibilities. For the next two years we would be placed in a variety of patient settings. Our class work would include studies in disease conditions. Courses included Nursing Care of Medical and Surgical Patients, Care of Children, Care of Communicable Diseases, Obstetrical Nursing, Nursery Care, Psychology, Psychiatric Nursing, Nursing History, Nutrition, and Ethics.

We rotated into these various patient areas and even had to go to other facilities for those kinds of patient experiences in specialty areas that our hospital did not offer. These off-campus rotations were called *affiliations*. We had three of these affiliations. But my next experience was still on our home campus with the more seriously ill medical and surgical patients. Finally, I was going to get to try out my *CAP*.

POST CAPPING PROMOTION

Following Capping, I was promoted to the evening shift under the supervision of a R.N. or a senior student nurse. On evenings there would be three-to-five Registered Nurses in the entire hospital. At least two would be on the Obstetrical/Nursery unit and one on Pediatrics. The other would be the Evening Supervisor, and her duties would be to cover the emergency room, call in the operating room staff in case of surgery, obtain drugs from the pharmacy, and be available, hopefully, for the charge person of the patient units, to give supervision and assistance as needed.

Private duty nurses would often be with the more acutely ill patients, as we did not have intensive care units. Should the family not be able to hire such a nurse, the floor nurse would have to attend to this patient as well.

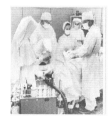

1947 Surgical team Rose de Lima Hospital Dignity Health St. Rose Dominican

76

Now keep in mind emergency rooms were not used back then for common illnesses but mainly for accidental and medical/surgical emergencies. In a small community hospital the case load on evening and night shifts was usually light. The supervisor made frequent rounds to each unit. In a small hospital we only had four medical-surgical units, and then the specialty units.

Upon arriving for our shift, we would hear a report on each patient from the day nurse who was ending her shift. The patients would be divided up between the students and the aids. The charge nurse would give all medicines and advanced treatments. The students would perform those procedures that they had learned so far, like taking blood pressures, giving enemas, etc. Every patient would get a backrub before bedtime. Oh, those were the days for the patients! Actually, we gave very good back massages. This luxury has long gone.

The shift was a busy one, but a good one to get to know your patients and their families. Answering lights, feeding patients, doing basic treatments, filling water pitchers, admitting new patients, and taking care of emergencies that might arise with patients kept us hopping. You see, a patient might have started bleeding, or a patient might have had an allergic reaction, or gone into insulin shock. You never knew what to expect, but you had to meet whatever challenge arose.

Patients who were having gastro examinations always had to have several enemas the night and morning before the examination. We did not have the gallon of cleansing liquid patients now have to drink that will accomplish the results that our enemas did back then. We did not have the three ounce disposable bowel cleansing plastic bottle we have today either. What we did have were the metal quart buckets and rubber tubing which came from Central Supply and had to be re-sterilized after use. Now, we had different types of enemas that the doctor could order. One was an S.S. or soapsuds enema. A second type was a mineral oil enema. The third was a three-H enema, which stood for *High, Hot and a H*** of a lot*, if you know what I mean.

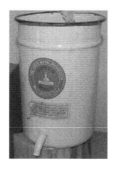

WWII-era bucket made by the Jonesware Metal Products Company.

After a week on this 3-11 shift, one became very proficient in executing this particular procedure. One of my classmates was assisting in giving the three-H enema and, while holding the bucket high, it tipped and the water dumped on top of her head, causing her cap to become soaked and limp. This was the same student who had to repeat the pledge three times.

While we younger students were busy doing the more basic procedures, the charge nurse was giving injections and medications and cleaning all the syringes and re-sterilizing them so they would be ready by the next three hour period, as most injections were given every three hours. A small electric sterilizer was in each medicine room.

Streptomycin and Penicillin, two fairly new miracle drugs, were now available to treat infections, and it seemed like almost every patient was getting these drugs. Again, we did not have the disposable syringes and needles. The charge nurse had to do most of the charting on every patient, too. We never even dreamed of computers. My word, television was just making its appearance. Yes, we had radios.

The position of the nurse with respect to the physician was one of following his orders and trying not to step over into the realm of practicing medicine. The physician was anxious to have the nurse's assistance as long as she knew her limits. For example, in charting or reporting on a patient, we nurses would say that the patient's dressing had "what appears to be an excessive amount of reddish-looking liquid," rather than "the patient is bleeding excessively". The latter would be defined as a nurse making a medical diagnosis. Goodness, that was a no-no! So we had to walk a fine line. It would be better to chart "the patient appears to have stopped breathing", rather than "patient has expired".

Now, I am just relating the way it was. While furthering my education in the late fifties and early sixties, I found an attitude of resistance from my doctor acquaintances to my effort to pursue this goal. However, nurses for the most part were just happy to nurse and, in fact, they

helped to deify the doctors and fed their egos. I was not
and am not anti-doctor; in fact, I have a son-in-law who
is a doctor. Still, women had their place, and all was well
as long as this situation did not change or be perceived
to be changing. This may sound exaggerated but,
honestly, I have tempered things considerably, as I did
not want to be tarred and feathered. Please do not kill
the messenger. I challenge any R.N. of my day to
correct me if I am exaggerating.

One day in the seventies as I was at my desk at a junior
college nursing program, a doctor I knew and respected
called me to tell me that the way we were now teaching
nursing was ruining nursing. You see, change is so
stressful for us humans. He was one who was like a
father figure to us as students. He was so kind, but he
liked the previous custom of having students on duty
around the clock. Students by this time were no longer
assigned to the evening or night shifts. How lucky for
them! It was a frustrating time for everyone caught in
these changing times.

It was, however, during this tour of duty that I
experienced my first death. This is something that is
never an event you want to observe. It is sobering and
emotional and stays with you for a while. We had to
prepare the body for the mortuary, which is not done by
nurses today, so I will not even go there. Fortunately,
the senior student assisted with this so I was not alone.
They say laughter and crying are finely related, and my
reaction under this stress was to suppress a nervous
sound between a giggle and a sob. We were to be brave

and not show our emotions by crying. Happily that thinking has changed over the years. One never gets used to death but you do handle it better as time passes. Your tears are often mixed with the families' tears, and that is okay.

You remember certain patients sometimes for the amusing things that happened. One patient was an elderly man who was foreign-born and he knew very little English. He was employed as a handy man for a family. It was Christmas and, feeling sorry for him, we students bought him a box of those chocolate-covered cherries, the cheapest kind, and gave it to him. You know, those that cause your teeth to ache the minute you open the box. At noon I took his meal tray into him and he took one look at the tray and rubbed his stomach and turned toward the wall and said, "No, no, no, seester!" I saw those little candy paper cups all over his bed and knew what had happened. Apparently he thought he had to eat the whole box at once. You see what miscommunication can do. He became so attached to us students, he cried when he had to leave.

It is now summer, 1948, and I am off for a month vacation. When I return, my next experience will be in Chicago, Illinois, at the Municipal Communicable Disease Hospital on California Avenue. Oh yes, polio was rampant and only diphtheria and smallpox had been controlled in this country. Tuberculosis patients were cared for in sanitariums. I had not a clue what I would experience in Chicago.

One year had now passed. I was not the same naïve, innocent young girl who started this journey a year ago. But one thing was for sure. This was truly my calling. Nursing was in my system, now, and the cap on my head felt like it was a perfect fit. I was one year closer to my goal.

DEAR GOD, I NEVER SIGNED UP FOR THIS!

Traveling to faraway places was not generally done by families in the forties. I had heard of Chicago, of course, and knew it was a big city adjacent to Lake Michigan in the northeastern part of our state. But the southern part of Illinois and the northern part of the state were two separate worlds; Chicago, and then Southern Illinois. Even in 1973 when, as a director of a nursing program, I invited my professional colleagues, while at a meeting in Chicago, to come downstate to our school for the next meeting. One nursing educator asked, "Well, how do we get there?" So you get the idea! Anyway, it is a great city and we students were so excited to go to the windy city.

An interesting bit of history about the start of Chicago was related to me while visiting Shawneetown, Illinois. This small town is located in southeastern Illinois, way down, almost over into Kentucky. It bordered the Ohio River, and one day some horseback riders came to town to ask to borrow money from one of the banks. This was for the purpose of starting this place we now know as Chicago. Ironically, the request was refused. The prevailing thought was that this place called Chicago would never amount to anything. Well, we all know the rest of this story.

Going to Chicago provided us with an opportunity to meet students from other schools and compare notes. Most of us came from similar small schools and when we first saw the immensity of the Municipal Contagious Disease Hospital, our mouths gaped open. The halls of one unit seemed to run on for a block. We were completely uninformed as to the nature of the illnesses we would encounter or the severity of the patient's conditions. I remember having had whooping cough (better known as Pertussis), measles, and chickenpox, and recall the quarantine sign placed on our house, so I thought I knew about contagious diseases. The coughing and choking I had with the whooping cough is still fresh in my memory.

During our orientation session it was stressed that strict isolation technique had to be maintained. This meant that we had to scrub up before we went into the patients' rooms and put on a mask and gown. When leaving the room we had to take off the gown and mask and scrub again. This same routine had to be done every time we went into another room to avoid what was known as cross-contamination. This meant if we broke technique then we might, for example, transfer measles to a child who already had another communicable disease. We were told that we students would be blamed if cross-contamination occurred. Well, this was a burden put upon us that we did not need. We already were scared for our lives. All other medical personnel went in and out of these rooms, also. Who could prove who had broken technique? This was the price for being the lowest on the totem pole.

The halls of each unit were built so that the small patient wards contained several beds lining each side of the unit. The wall nearest the hallway was a half-glass window panel. This made the patients visible to those parents who had to remain isolated from them in the glassed corridors in the middle of the hallway. Outside these glassed-in corridors were the hallways the nurses could use to go in and out of the rooms and up and down the hall. Since the majority of the patients were children, parents standing confined in these hallways found it quite traumatic not to be able to hold or talk with their sick or possibly dying child.

Many of the children came from very poor living conditions and were malnourished. Not only did they have communicable diseases but with low resistance to infection, they were very seriously ill with complications like pneumonia, ear infections, and meningitis. Pertussis usually was accompanied by pneumonia in these children and they required frequent suctioning of thick mucus from the throat. In the front of the long halls of these units were suctioning rooms that had once been used for diphtheria patients. Now they were mainly for pertussis children. The suctioning tubes were fastened to water faucets in a way that a suction action was produced. Yes, it was archaic, but the best we had, and it served the purpose.

Quite frequently, when caring for these children, we would have to pick up a youngster, rush down the hall with a choking child, and pray that we made it to the suction room in time. At times a tracheotomy would have to be done if the edema (swelling) and mucus had caused respiratory distress. So young we were, and yet the responsibilities were so great.

Children who developed meningitis were gravely ill and as the disease progressed, their heads would hyperextend and their feet and lower extremities would bend upward toward the back of their head. This was called an opisthotonos position. Treatment for these severe infections consisted of injections of Streptomycin and Penicillin in large doses. However, such dosages would cause deafness. These drugs only came into use during World War II, so prior to this time we had no antibiotics to combat such infections. The death rate was high in those days.

These types of patients were quite a challenge for us young novices. We were assigned to an eight-hour shift either on days, evenings, or nights. We students were responsible to the charge nurse or other staff members. Some whom we worked with were very helpful while others were not. The seriousness of our patients' conditions and the feelings of being ill-equipped to assume such responsibilities were overwhelming. Leaving our shift of duty and returning to our dormitory rooms, we often threw ourselves onto the bed and cried, feeling that this tour of duty would never end.

The most stressful experience for me was caring for polio patients. The thought of getting polio ourselves was frightening as it was caused by a virus. There were two types of polio. One was called Bulbar Polio, which paralyzed the throat and respiratory muscles. The other type affected the spinal cord and caused paralysis of the upper and lower extremities.

In the earlier stage of the disease we could distinguish the type by the presenting symptoms. A child would come in with early suspicion of polio and within hours, if the child took a drink of milk or water and the fluid came back out of the nose, we knew he most likely had Bulbar Polio. That indicated paralysis of the throat and upper respiratory muscles and the child would be rushed to the iron lung room. I don't have the words to describe to you the true nature of this disease.

These large iron lung receptacles looked like a tank with portholes on the sides so we nursing personnel could put our hands and arms through these apertures to care for the patient. Only the child's head was out of the tank. The tank had to be airtight and create a negative pressure so the respiratory muscles could rise and fall as the rubber bellows below rose up and down, making a constant rhythmic "whoosh". Several tanks would be in one large room. The parents were lined up out in the glassed in corridors watching, praying, crying, and grieving for their child. The young children fought for their lives and often frustration built up and the only way they had to express their fear and dread of confinement in this scary machine was to try and "spit".

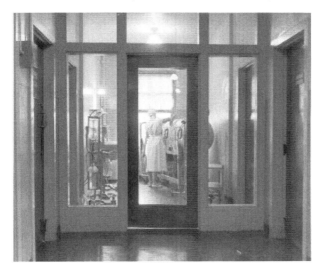

Iron Lung BJC Healthcare Pinterest page historic Alton Hospital photos

Notes would be written and sent to us by the parents so we could read them to these children. "Tommy," one said, "Hang in there, son. Mother and Daddy love you so much. We are praying to Jesus that you will be well soon so we can take you home. We are just outside in the hall and we can see you and we will be here. Let the nurses do what they have to do for now, O.K.? Love, Mommy and Daddy."

Years later, when my two children were born, I would look at them and then look up to God and say a prayer of thanks for the development of the polio vaccine, knowing that my children and others would never have to fear this disease (I pray not). To also have the immunizations for the other childhood contagious diseases made us parents so blessed.

But then, my feelings would range from anger to grief as we watched so many children either die or have serious, debilitating paralysis. And it did not help to live in fear of becoming ill ourselves due to our contact with these patients. "What am I doing here and how much longer is this tour of duty? Oh, God, I want to go home. I never signed up for this! Why, why, do these children have to suffer like this? Maybe I am not really cut out for this profession! These kids need help!". Help did eventually arrive, but not in time to save many of these children. Additional childhood immunizations and the polio vaccine had yet to emerge upon the health scene. Bless all of you researchers, and especially you, Dr. Salk.

Physical therapy was a big part of the care of these children who had damage to the nerves and muscles. The use of hot packs and muscle exercises were part the nurses' duty, as this was prior to the emergence of the physical therapist. It was because of polio that the need for such a therapist was recognized. Nurses became a little concerned when both physical therapist and respiratory therapist came on the scene. It was seen as if some of our duties were being taken away. But the value of these therapists was soon recognized as a blessing to us and especially the patients.

Before we ended our time in Chicago, we had to make some house calls to some of these children's homes. Chicago, like many other big cities, had its areas where, of course, living conditions were deplorable. The smell of urine, vomit and alcohol and the Lord knows what else, are nauseating odors that one never forgets. I often look back and think, "Great! Sending us out into those districts was not safe for many reasons." I try not to ponder the possible consequences of those assignments. Learning how others had to live was an eye opener, though.

Fortunately, Chicago offered many attractions for us to take in during our free times and help us forget for a day or two the misery of the hospital situation. The museums, the zoo, the lake, the theaters, and the fresh air enabled us to survive. This entire experience has stayed with me and I know now why at 18, I felt much, much older and yes, wiser. If you think this experience was a little much, hang on a little longer.

Wait until I tell you about living on the grounds of a mental institution for my three months of experience in Psychiatric Nursing. Oh, yes, if ever you have seen *One Flew Over the Cuckoo's Nest* then you will be able to relate somewhat to what it must have been like.

As we rode the train back down to southern Illinois, we felt that we had aged quite a bit. We had experienced too much of suffering and death. It seems to hurt more when children are involved. We had seen poverty like we had never known. We saw life in a different way. We looked forward to getting back to our small community and families and our small hospital home up on such a scenic, peaceful hill. Such a contrast!

BEHIND CLOSED, LOCKED DOORS

Some say the times in which we live define us. We are born into a particular time and become a part of it, the good and the bad. Each generation has to deal with the bad and accept things as they are, or make the needed changes to lessen the bad. Often changes cannot be made until new inventions come along, or new discoveries are made in the medical world, like the Salk vaccine that we talked about earlier.

Some changes occur only when people make attitude changes and remove prejudices and other injustices. No generation is born into an ideal society so, critical as we may be about past generations, we had better look around and see where our own weaknesses still lie, knowing the next generations might question, perhaps, even our humanity.

This leads to my next affiliation, which was the psychiatric experience in a mental hospital found in the middle of our great state, in Jacksonville, Illinois. There was no preparation for this kind of duty for if we really knew what lay ahead I am afraid the dropout rate in nursing schools would have been much higher than it was. Each of us had our own perception of the mentally ill. Words like crazy, loco, nutty, psycho, etc., were among the words we heard used.

The many psychotropic drugs used today were not realized, as yet. The behavior modification treatments used were heavy sedatives like Choral Hydrate, isolation, mummy wraps of cold sheets, recreational and occupational activities, and, oh yes, electric shock, and in extreme cases, brain lobotomy and induced insulin shock.

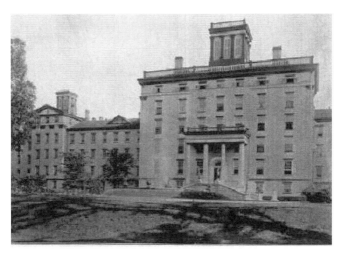

Jacksonville State Hospital, from the Illinois State Archives

I can just imagine your shock and dismay, but later, in the sixties our society supposedly did all these people a favor by shutting down these institutions. The clients transferred out into our city streets, and they now make up a majority of what we call homeless people. A more humane method, you think? Hmm! And only a few years earlier our country had allowed mass sterilizations of so called "mental" individuals. In reality, the plan, in

1963 under the Kennedy administration, had been for
the communities to set up homes or some safe havens
where these clients would find placement and treatment.
That never materialized as planned, and many of these
individuals fell through the cracks.

We can be grateful, though, for many of the new
psychiatric drugs, to be sure. These allow many patients
to be able to function quite well in society. Others are in
nursing homes or able to live independently with
welfare assistance. And then there are those who fall
through the cracks and live under our bridges. The
homeless mentally ill are still a problem that we have
not totally solved as yet.

But this was 1948 and students lived on the grounds of
the hospital that was surrounded by high iron fences
with locked gates. We entered the doors of the hospital
and they were locked behind us. The type of patients, or
clients, as we now call them, were as follows: Manic
depressive or bi-polar, schizophrenia, suicidal, violent,
catatonic, drug addictions, vegetative, and syphilitic
brain disorder.

Patients who heard voices became very agitated at
times, even arguing with the voices or striking out at
them. Some were not aware of reality and reasoning
with them was in vain. Some were living in Bible times
and would tell you, for example, as they would quote
scripture, "not to step on the mantle that had been laid
down at the door." Taking away their Bible for a time
would be indicated while they were in this state of mind,
an action which people of faith sometimes did not

understand. These patients were so obsessed with some idea from the Bible that letting them have their Bibles just prolonged the obsession. The clergy and psychologist were not supportive of each other then, but better relations seem to exist today. Spiritual care is very important in any kind of patient situation.

Other patients would stay in one position as if in a stupor, trance-like, neglecting nutrition, hygiene, and other normal, daily activities. Those who became violent would be placed in isolation or be heavily sedated for a time. Those who had agitation depression would pace constantly. Those who were saddened by depression would be inactive and often verbalize suicidal ideas. Three months of this atmosphere was our fate.

To make us know how the client felt, we had to personally endure some of these treatments, like being rolled up in ice sheets in a mummy-like fashion. Now, that is a feeling for you. Being tightly and snugly wrapped so you cannot move causes your heart rate to increase dramatically, and you reach the point of feeling panicky. The effect was to be one of calming the person but to me it did the opposite. I thought, "Oh, if my parents could see me now!" And "Oh, my! What if a fire breaks out?"

It took us a while to be able to recognize mental illness in some patients. I remember talking to a nice, mid-sixties-aged man. We had the sanest conversation until he began to tell me about his neighbor, Abraham Lincoln. Our class work did help us to know how to relate to these patients without agitating them.

One of the methods used as treatment, electric shock, is still used today but only minimally for deep depression that has not responded to medicine, and especially for patients who pose a high risk for suicide. The method is nothing like it was in 1948. It is done under mild anesthesia and the seizure resulting is like a mild tremor of a toe. Would I recommend it today? Yes. But only if the doctor felt this was probably a life-saving measure due to poor response to antidepressants. However, as a student I had to assist many times with the old method and it was not pleasant. We had to restrain the client and it would take about four of us to hold firmly onto the client's extremities at the joints to prevent injury during the *grand mal* seizure produced by the electric current.

Remember, the doctor was limited in his choice of treatments that would help in extreme cases. Today most clients can be treated in a Psychiatric Unit in a medical hospital, receive an effective drug regimen and psychotherapy, and have follow-up care at home by social services. Electric shock is used in very selective cases.

Our classwork in this experience was very helpful in understanding what we were dealing with, but the clinical experience was really emotionally taxing. For the most part, of course, these clients were not confined to beds, so care was not as physical. We gave medications, assisted in treatments already mentioned, went to recreational therapy, played cards or ping-pong. Occupational therapy consisted of crafts and learning life and social skills. Because of the lack of medicines that lift patients out of depression or change erratic and/or violent behavior, these clients were imprisoned, so to speak, and kept away from society. But would we, today, have done any better with these clients under the same circumstances?

The social stigma in our country toward mental illness was one of misunderstanding, or one might even say ignorance, disdain, and ridicule. I would like to think we have overcome that stigma, but not completely. Many people are still reluctant to admit the need to obtain professional help out of shame and because of fear of what others will say. Many will resist admitting they are depressed or suffering from anxiety or stress and will keep trying to find physical reasons for the condition. We still have a long way to go in educating the public, but thank goodness strides have been made. I am grateful that today's student nurse does not have to go through some of those experiences in psychiatric nursing as we did in 1948.

PEDIATRIC NURSING AFFILIATION

Our third affiliation was to take place in Children's Memorial Hospital on Fullerton Ave. in Chicago, Ill. This was and still is a well-known hospital. This experience was more bearable than the time we spent on California Avenue at the Contagious Disease

Hospital. We rotated among specialty units like the heart unit, the orthopedic unit, the surgical and medical units. Our classroom work covered the diseases affecting children and their nursing care.

It was another experience where we cared for critically-ill children. At times it was difficult, but we were third year students now, a little bit more capable of seeing the suffering in children. I do remember one evening working on the Orthopedic Unit and having a young boy who was in a body cast jump on my back and knock me to the floor. He was just being playful. One three-year-old boy who had both legs broken and was lying with his legs up in the air in traction. When asked how he was injured, would say, "Oh, my daddy did this." In reality, he and his dad were playing and the father swung him by his legs, injuring both legs. This was a rather fun and easy unit.

I was impressed by the nursing and medical staff at this hospital. It always has had a good reputation, and we did see and learn a lot while there. Pediatric nursing is very rewarding, especially when you see the children happily go home with their parents. On the other hand, the most difficult aspect is dealing with the death of a child.

When I returned home and worked in the Pediatric unit, the most memorable thing was the fact that the parents could only see their child during limited visiting hours. Those were the rules and they were enforced. Thankfully, today, that is not the case, nor would parents stand for such a rule. It was like the moment you put your child in the unit he or she was not yours anymore. This was traumatic to parents and the child. I remember once my three-year-old was hospitalized and after leaving in obedience to the strict visiting hour rule, my husband Ron and I sat in the lobby and cried as we heard our daughter cry after us. Today, most parents stay with their child, and in fact it is welcomed.

THE SCRUB NURSE

My rotation to the operating room was next on my schedule; an experience that I was not fondly looking forward to. I was rather intimidated by the surgeons and, to work next to them in surgery, frankly, frightened me. I had heard about some who threw temper tantrums. Some might throw an instrument across the room, and other horror stories. I never witnessed this behavior. Yes, some were God-like and temperamental, but others were very well-mannered and walked us through the procedure, helping us to learn anatomy and physiology.

We had to learn all the names of the instruments and be able to hand them to the doctor when he asked for them. Learning to scrub, gown-and-glove-up, and knowing how to keep a field sterile, were top priorities in surgery. Counting of the sponges before the surgeon closed the wound was an exercise that was very important. The count had to be the same as that which you had counted before the operation took place. Once in a while the doctor would hide one, just checking to see if we came up with one missing. A missing sponge could indicate that one had been left inside the patient.

If this experience of assisting with operations did nothing else, it made our generation of nurses very aware of the importance of sterile technique. I cringe today at what I see that is supposed to be sterile technic by some medical personnel. I am sorry but it is not the same. Could this be one of the reason why Staph infections occur more readily nowadays? Just wondering.

OBSTETRICAL/NURSERY NURSING

We all looked forward to seeing babies born and caring for these infants.

This meant we would be with women during their labor and delivery and also spend time working in the nursery. My first assignment was to be with the mother in the labor room and this could be for a brief time or prolonged labor time. The labor nurse would do the examinations on the women to see how dilated the cervix was, which would give us an inkling of when the baby was to be delivered. The students were supposed to learn how to do this procedure as well, but I never became proficient and never intended to become an obstetrical nurse.

Timing the contractions was part of our responsibility, as was keeping the husband informed. Husbands were not allowed in the delivery room. They were left to pace in a separate room. It was not until the 1960s that husbands were permitted to be in the delivery room. It is so great that fathers can be part of the delivery experiences today. Even the whole neighborhood is welcomed. Just kidding!

When the cervix was about fully dilated, the doctor would be called and occasionally the physician did not make it in time. The nurse, not the student, had to deliver the baby. I do recall that the patient received ether as an anesthetic. The delivery of a healthy baby was a very joyous occasion. This was the fun part. There is nothing like seeing the parents loving on a newly born baby. I did not, however, have much patience with a father who cried because the baby was not a boy.

Caesarean sections were done in surgery and I liked to assist with these as the baby's head was beautifully shaped. Coming through the birth canal often causes a misshaping of the newborn head. My first was a daughter and her nose was smashed as if she had been in boxing ring. In spite of that, my husband would put her picture under people's noses and say, "Isn't that the most beautiful baby you ever saw?"

The stay in the hospital for mothers was much longer than it is today, as it was for most other kinds of patients. Postpartum care lasted five days barring complications. The mother was given classes in how to care for her baby before going home. Since this was before rooming-in of the infant, all of the babies were in the nursery and carried out to the mother at feeding times. Any baby who was critically ill was cared for in a separate nursery and in many cases sent to a larger hospital where the infants would have specialized care. Thank goodness, we now have neonatal intensive care units.

Many of you may not know of this fact, but oxygen was often given at a high concentration level to babies in distress, especially premature infants. This was a factor in causing blindness in these children, something that wasn't known at the time. The procedure that was modified when it was determined this oxygen level was the culprit. I had a classmate that had a daughter that was a victim of this method of treatment. Learning often has a price!

PRE-GRADUATION TOUR OF DUTY

Being senior students meant that one would most likely be placed on a unit as a charge person on evenings or nights, along with an aid or two. I was placed on a unit with medical, surgical, and orthopedic conditions. When assigned to the night shift, I would report for duty at 11:00 p.m. and receive a report on the patients by the nurse who was on evenings. I would make my rounds, checking on the patients. This would take about an hour and then I would return to the medicine room and prepare my medications for the 12:00 time. After giving the medicines, I would return to the medicine room, rinse the needles and syringes, and put them into a sterilizer to get them ready for the 3:00 a.m. medicine rounds. I would also repeat this at 6 a.m.

I would check the temperatures and blood pressure readings of the patients taken by the aid. Any patient having surgery the next day would have to be placed on fasting from food and water. This was referred to by NPO, meaning nothing by mouth. Enemas would have to be given to them in the early morning. For those who were receiving intravenous fluids, we would have to see if the needle was still in the vein and not leaking, or infiltrating, as it was called. Dressings would have to be checked to be sure no one was bleeding excessively. We had to empty and turn over the Wangonsteen stomach suction bottles, checking circulation of the skin of cast patients, and so on. Sometimes a new patient would have to be admitted and a physician called for orders during the other routine things going on.

When time afforded itself one would have to chart on all of the patients. Meanwhile, the aid would be answering bed call lights and reporting to you those things that needed the nurse's attention. With medicines being needed every three hours and the in-between activities, the night goes very quickly. Should there be a major problem or concern, the night R.N. supervisor was called for assistance and advice.

Early morning became very active with preparing the surgical patients and giving morning care to all the patients. At 7:00 a.m., the day staff appeared and was ready for a report on the patients' conditions. Whew! A long night!

As I charted my last notation on my last night in school, my emotions were mixed. There was sadness at leaving what had been my home for three years; the closeness of the medical and nursing staff; the memory of so many patients who taught me so much, and yet, excitement at what lay ahead. Little did I know the career opportunities that would come my way, built upon the knowledge and skills I gained in this small community Diploma nursing program? It was just the start of my educational and career pursuit, but what a start.

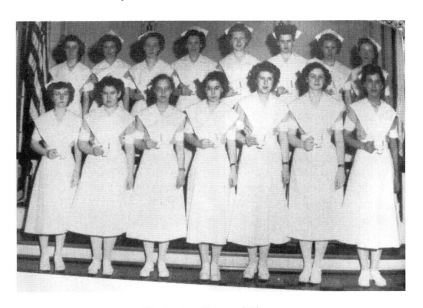

Graduation Personal Photo

THE DIPLOMA NURSE: HER SHINING DAY, HER FADING TOUCH
The Heart Cry of a Nurse

Dear Lord, the night was long, and I am so tired.
The patients were restless and some were wired.
The call lights were numerous; too many to please.
I only wanted to put them at ease.

The look on some showed hopelessness and fear
They wanted to talk, so I stayed near
I held their hand and wiped their brow
And asked, "Can I do more, and how?"

The hard part came when at one bed I knew
A life was ending, not a thing I could do
But comfort the family and whisper a prayer
And thank the Lord that I was there.

For being there was my call
When I opted to walk those halls
To offer a smile and open my heart
Were gifts God gave me from the start

Though I may complain and whine away
You note that I decided to stay
For my rewards outshine silver or gold
A new day a new patient a new story unfolds

So Lord, don't you mind when I complain
I really don't mean to be such a pain
For nursing is my life, my love, my all
For the least of these, I obeyed your call.

Jessie Wilson, 2012

Part V Notations on an Amazing Journey

Some critics found the time we spent in clinical experience as only repetition of things already learned. I would agree with that about the technical skills, but nursing is more than technical procedures. Each exposure to a new patient presents new learning opportunities as each patient responds differently to illness. Your observation and communication skills are put to the test and are strengthened. Our organizational skills enabled us to be more efficient. We can liken this experience to an orientation program today, perhaps, for it did give us confidence upon entering into the work setting following graduation. Some may call this free labor for the hospital, but it certainly paid off for us.

Is it no wonder we students could walk out of the doors of the hospital and be ready to step into the shoes and function as a clinically-skilled Registered Nurse upon passing our state boards? Upon graduation we were given a gold pin to wear, and ours was designed after the doors of our hospital. The pin identified the nursing school that we had attended. We wore the pin proudly. We knew the blood and sweat it had cost us but, no regrets. Pinning ceremonies are often held today to present these pins to the graduating nursing class.

The debate over whether the learning style of the Diploma nurse was right or wrong should now be a moot issue. Her contribution to nursing for the past sixty years has been indisputable and is a testimony to the young woman of this era and her capability to meet the challenge of her day, just as Florence Nightingale did before her. Florence did not have ideal conditions either. So to this Diploma Nurse, let us take our caps off (figuratively speaking), be grateful, and see that the history of nursing gives this nurse her due.

May today's student nurse, also, be made of just the right stuff for the challenges faced in a totally different nursing practice world. May she love her profession as much, and still believe it can be a worthy calling from God. May she recognize the importance of her *touch* to a patient.

Even though the nursing cap is not a required part of a dress code, and though you, the new nurses, have the needed knowledge and are hopefully given the needed time to develop clinical competency, may you realize it is your core being, your heart, and your own DNA that distinguishes your *touch* from all others. It always has been and always will be! That is your gift that you bring to your profession.

We Diploma nurses pass the mantle on to you, the modern degree nurse. Wear it proudly and with dignity so our story will not be in vain. Appreciate the legacy which paved the way for your day.

There are not many of these Diploma nurses that I have highlighted in this story still living, but when two or three of them get together in a room, they may be strangers to each other, but something draws one nurse to another, and their conversation turns to those days they cherished so long ago. They exchange stories and completely exclude all others in the room. They know they nursed in a unique day and in a unique way. And they were right for that time! Would they want those days to come back? Hardly! Were they proud of the job they did? Most assuredly!

I know God gave me further affirmation that my opinion of this nurse is not off-base. I recently had a colonoscopy and a young LPN assisted me for this procedure. We, of course, discussed nursing. I told him of the story I was writing. He said, "I have worked with nurses that graduated from St. John's School of Nursing here in Tulsa, and they are great nurses." I whispered to myself, "Thank you, Kevin, and thank you, Lord. I needed that!" Yes, there is a difference about those nurses.

Like old soldiers, our touch will *fade* but never die. Florence Nightingale paved the way before us and we have kept her lamp **flickering,** through every patient we have cared for or nursing student we have taught. Though in my senior years, now, these memories are as real to me as if they happened yesterday. Thanks for re-living my journey with me.

Part VI From Diploma Nurse to Degree Nurse Educator – Passing the Touch to the Modern Generation.

"I QUIT, LORD. IF YOU HAVE ANY MINISTRY FOR ME, PLEASE BRING IT TO ME. AMEN."

The following shows how God can use an average person like me when we surrender to Him and let Him chart our course. I was not a person who seemed capable of facing the huge challenges the Lord brought into my life. I was socially introverted, had very little self-esteem, was compliant, nonassertive, and non-confrontational. I lived in an era when it was not the thing for women to work outside the home, nor to be assertive.

I prayed the above prayer in 1970. I was discouraged with teaching in the late sixties and early seventies. The students were too restless to focus on nursing studies.

They focused on protesting the Vietnam War. Some became Flower Children. The use of LSD was an issue. How can you teach people how to care for other human beings when the students are not "in the mood"? One colleague looked at me and said, "you know, we are too good for these students. They don't deserve us."

I said, "You know, you are right. I am going to go home and work in my flower garden." And so I did just that.

I was not at home very long when an opportunity to be the Director at St. Mary's Hospital in East St. Louis came my way. East St. Louis was known then as a low-income area with mostly black residents where a million dollars a day poured into the city from the government to help the citizens. However, it seemed it never got down to the people it was designated for. Of course not!

I had to drive about 30 miles to work so it was not convenient. Little did I know God would teach me some needed lessons for down the road. In about twelve months he would have another place already picked out for me. In the meantime, I got an education that prepared me for what was still to come; a streetwise education.

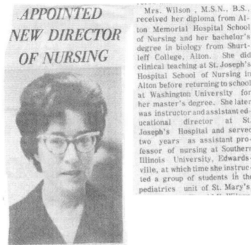

APPOINTED NEW DIRECTOR OF NURSING

Mrs. Wilson, M.S.N., B.S., received her diploma from Alton Memorial Hospital School of Nursing and her bachelor's degree in biology from Shurtleff College, Alton. She did clinical teaching at St. Joseph's Hospital School of Nursing in Alton before returning to school at Washington University for her master's degree. She later was instructor and assistant educational director at St. Joseph's Hospital and served two years as assistant professor of nursing at Southern Illinois University, Edwardsville, at which time she instructed a group of students in the pediatrics unit of St. Mary's.

Mrs. Jessie M. Wilson

"I have a philosophy about nursing", said Mrs. Jessie M. Wilson who has been appointed director of nursing service of St. Mary's Hospital, East St. Louis. "I think nursing has to get back to the patient. Skilled nurses have been letting themselves get tied down with too much paper work and have let other personnel perform duties that nurses are best suited to perform. They have become more of an administrator and less of a practitioner. I am optimistic, however, that at St. Mary's, we are going to reverse this situation".

It was a city where it was not safe to be on the streets at night. When some of my night nurses would tell me they needed to be on days so they would not have to leave their children at home at night by themselves, I would listen and make better arrangements for them. It was a place where on occasion I had to put security around some of my nursing stations to protect my nursing staff. One day the police had a hot pursuit after

110

a person through the hospital halls. Thank goodness I had some fine nuns around me who had me in their prayers. I kept them on their knees.

I had, in the short time that I was there, one unit which did not want to be co-operate with the policies of the hospital, so the staff called a blue flustrike. Everyone called in sick, leaving the poor head nurse all by herself, acting innocently, as if she were not a part of the problem, when in fact she was leading it.

If you think I was prepared for all of this you are totally wrong. I did a lot of praying, believe me! I met the head nurse at 6 a.m one morning and she and her cohort, a medical man, were there all by themselves. So I sort of addressed myself to both of them. They were so taken aback they just stood there, shell-shocked. A maintenance man who was a Christian stood by. He pulled me aside and said, "Wow, they looked like the lions in Daniel's Den with taped up mouths." I had made rounds during the night and had talked to the staff to see if this strike was spreading. It was not, so that gave me the strength to confront the issue. Fortunately, the matter soon was resolved, by way of a new head nurse.

The challenges I had in this experience paid off in my later positions. A big task that was also facing me was the dedication of a new Intensive Care Unit. When it had been completed, the public relations man, whose office was across from mine, wanted to make a big deal out of this event. He called the White House to ask President Nixon to come and be a part of the dedication. You see, a lot of politics was tied into this city. Everyone wanted to get the praise for "helping the poor". Yes, indeed. Well, instead of the president, we got Senator Ted Kennedy.

On the day before and the day of the dedication, we had secret service men all over the hospital and surrounding area. On the big night I had to go down and give permission for my husband to come into the hospital. The crowd in the hospital was huge. Senator Kennedy and I and the head nurse were the only three allowed in the intensive care unit while pictures were being taken. The local newspaper had a field day with this event. It was quite an experience.

I was responsible for 325 staff employees and filled in for the administrator when he was gone. This administration was not engaged in the nursing issues nor did he want to be bothered too much. Contact between my office and the administrator was minimal. This bothered me quite a bit, but it was part of the culture still, in my opinion, of not valuing women in leadership, and wanting nursing to be there as long as we kept in our place and didn't cause trouble.

JESSIE GLOVER WILSON

ALTON TELEGRAPH   Wed., March 2, 1977   A-3

L&C nursing program accredited

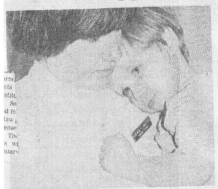

Lewis & Clark Community College has recently obtained accreditation from the National League for Nursing (NLN) for the College's Associate Degree Nursing Program, President Wilbur R. L. Trimpe has announced.

The accreditation is voluntary and beyond the minimal requirements for operating a nursing program. Seeking and being granted accreditation brings national recognition to the school and points out the quality of the nursing staff and the program they present.

According to the NLN, accreditation, while being important in helping to recruit outstanding faculty to teach at Lewis & Clark, is also an important and beneficial factor to the students. NLN statistics show that graduates of accredited programs have a better chance of passing the all-important state licensure examinations which permit them to practice as registered nurses.

The accreditation of the Associate Degree Nursing Program is the third health care program at Lewis and Clark Community College to obtain national recognition. The Medical Laboratory Technician Program is accredited by the American Medical Association Council on Medical Education through the National Accreditation Agency for Clinical Laboratory Sciences.

Student nurse, Beverly LeMaster (above) of Edwardsville, with pensive patient, Sue Hyman (below) of Shipman, student, gives a hairdo.

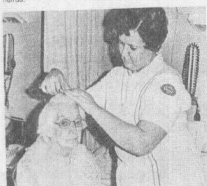

KATHY GARDNER talks to patient.

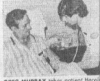

GREG MURRAY takes patient Harold Eberlin's blood pressure.

My favorite part of this experience was working with
the nursing staff, and, even though most of them were
non-Caucasian, we got along well. I admired them
because they were hard-working individuals just trying
to make a living. But just as I was settling in, I had a
visit from a college administrator from my home town
who asked me to come and direct a new Associate
Degree program at the Lewis and Clark Community
College in Godfrey, Illinois. There had been some
birthing problems with this program and because this
was my home town, I could now see why God had me
out of the local situation during this time. It removed
me from the politics so I could come in clean and with
an open mind, so to speak.

I knew that I could not do much more to improve the
situation here in East St. Louis, considering the lack of a
close working relationship with administration, so I was
interested in this new position. Teaching was my
passion, anyway. After all, I had told the Lord to come
after me when He had a job for me to do. I left St.
Mary's knowing I had gained the respect of the
employees. The nuns were great to work with but it
appeared they had little clout in this situation. The
public relations man, in a letter of reference, was
complimentary, and remarked that I was a woman to be
respected, and most of all "a lady". God had me there
for a purpose, probably more for my benefit than

anything else. I had never been close to this culture and I found it was good for me. I changed many of my preconceived ideas, learned to love the people, and observed the strength and courage many of them had trying to live under difficult circumstances. I was a better person for having had this opportunity.

HOMETOWN BECKONS

Lewis and Clark Community College had formerly been an all-girls' college but had been converted into a Junior College. Both Schools of Nursing, Alton Memorial Hospital and St. Joseph Hospital, had been forced to close because of the young men and women entering nursing in the seventies now wanting a degree program.

This was hard for this community to accept so I knew there would be plenty of critics to contend with. The newspaper had carried the struggles of the school, public meetings were held, and there were pros and cons to the situation, so townspeople took sides. The students took sides as well. It was my job to get this situation calmed down. I had gone to school at Alton Memorial Hospital myself and had taught at both of these community diploma programs. Only God could

have arranged for me to now be involved and have this
opportunity to get this new Associates Degree program
on a firm foundation.

Of course, there was the job of completing the nursing
faculty. The director can never do the job alone. Some I
had taught with before. Others were new to me.

A pattern was beginning to occur for me. "Lord," I said,
"Now why are you putting me in places that are going
to be difficult?" This was now 1972. More and more
diploma schools were becoming Associate Degree
programs. This meant part of the community, especially
the medical community, was not going to be happy with
this development. I got static from students who had
taken sides in whatever the problem had been, and from
the doctors, and some older Diploma nurses who, of
course, were loyal to the Diploma schools. I understood
all of this. Since students were still in a rebellious state
in this country, any excuse they could find to cause an
uprise, they jumped on the bandwagon. But God had
put me there, and so my reliance upon him was my
rock.

I had a strong faculty and we got to work to see to it
that we had a quality program. Within three years we
were able to obtain national accreditation for the
program from the National League of Nursing. The
accreditor who examined our program asked me why

we had tried so soon to obtain this accreditation. I told her we had to quickly prove to the community that we had a nursing program that not only met the standards for the State of Illinois, but also those of the national accrediting board. The percentage of passing rate on the Registered Nurse exams ranged between 98 to 99 percent.

Hannibal Courier-Post   Tuesday, June 28, 1988

Nurses program gets accreditation

Hannibal-LaGrange College's Associate Degree Nursing Program will be granted an initial accreditation status, the college has learned.

Cyndi Allison, public relations director for the college, announced Wednesday that the status was granted this month in New York City by a panel of Associate Degree nurse educators from the National League for Nursing.

Criteria studied by the panel before granting the accreditation included a review of an in-depth self-evaluation study that was submitted to the NLN by the nursing faculty at the college. Criteria also included a favorable report by two site visitors from the NLN, and an interview between Dr. Sandra Stevenson of Troy State University, Montgomery, Ala., and Jessie Wilson, director of nurses at H-LG.

The college's nursing program has been accredited by the Missouri State Board of Nursing since October 1980.

Wilson said, "This additional accreditation status from the NLN is a voluntary accreditation that carries with it an accountability to nursing, education and consumers. The students that enter the ADN program will now have a greater assurance that the program is considered to be a quality program."

Wilson said the changed status will give students "a greater sense of security that they can continue to build upon when they go on to further their education. Some universities and colleges make it a requirement that incoming ADN students have graduated from a NLN accredited institution."

Current H-LG nursing faculty members Edie Daniel, Lisa Haschemeyer, Cindy Riley and Karin Baughman assisted Wilson in the project.

Review of the accreditation will be made at eight-year intervals.

I remained in this position until the spring of 1980 and had a feeling that God was up to something again. Spring is a hard time on campus. It is testing time, graduation time, and a time to get resignations from faculty. I had a rough night sleeping the right before Good Friday. I wrestled in my bed and finally prayed, "Lord, I need a sign of what you want me to do."

The next morning I walked into my office, and my phone was ringing. It was Dr. Brown, Vice-President of Hannibal-La Grange College, a conservative Southern Baptist Bible college. "We have been given the money to have nursing program and your name was recommended by a former student of yours."

I would not have been considered for this job had my husband and I not recently joined a Southern Baptist church. I quickly said that I was not interested. The distance was 100 miles from our home. He asked me to pray about it. *Great!* I called my husband Ron and told him. He said, without pausing, "When the Lord opens a door; you had better check it out." I am sure you can see where this is going.

So, on Good Friday, Ron and I made our way up the west side of Illinois by way of a very scenic road to Mark Twain's old home grounds. The task at hand, as Dr. Brown explained, was that the facility for the nursing school had to be designed and furnished; a curriculum developed; faculty hired, and approval obtained from the State Board of Nursing. That was all! I visited the two hospitals that they would be using for clinical labs to see how they felt about this program.

Here was an opportunity for me to serve with a Christian college. It was inviting, but my husband and I had to work out some issues. He worked at McDonnell Douglas Aircraft Corporation, 100 miles away. So after consulting with our Lord we both felt that this was an opportunity for me. I accepted this challenge on the basis that I would commute for a year, get it started, and then determine whether we could remain or not. Both of our children were in college so they posed no problem.

I had a room in the faculty residence to stay overnight from time to time. The community did need the program as they had a shortage of nursing staff. In addition, the young men and women of the area who wanted a nursing career needed the program because frankly, the area was not wealthy. Most young people could not afford to travel to a distant college or university to acquire a nursing education.

Hannibal, according to a book written about it called "White Town Drowsing", was a little slower in getting with the times. An outsider or stranger was viewed with suspicion. In fact, as of 1983 you could find small churches in the area that still had men sitting on one side and women on the other. I kid you not. Once people got to know you it was a friendly town. Its tourist attraction, of course, was Mark Twain's home. Indeed, that did bring in the tourists. Located on the Mississippi, it is a very beautiful, scenic area.

The only place the school had for the nursing lab was in the basement of the Science building. Believe it or not I had to design the lab, classrooms, instructors' office areas, personally buy the furnishings, and at the same time develop the curriculum from scratch. All this was on a limited budget. The school was on shaky financial ground and salaries were unbelievably low, but most of the faculty were dedicated Christians who were willing to work for these salaries. The school had been known for just being a Bible college but now they wanted to expand with secular programs. I knew that when they brought in such secular programs, better salaries would have to be paid. That proved to be accurate. And it enabled the older faculty to upgrade their status, which they dearly deserved.

I had learned by now to be more assertive and as I look back I guess I came off aggressive to these pastors. After all, women then in most Baptist churches were to be submissive, and certainly not assertive. I was raised like that. But by now I was beginning to wonder if my assertiveness was going to be a problem, because passivity would not get us to where we needed to go in this situation. Doesn't the Lord have a sense of humor?

Their policies for faculty required that faculty be Southern Baptist. Well, I understood the school wanting nursing instructors that were Christians but also the instructors needed the academic degrees necessary for them to teach nursing. I was willing to settle for a Christian of another denomination if she/he had the academic qualifications. So I advertised all over the country and did not find any one who wanted to come to the rural area of Hannibal, Missouri. With the opening of school approaching, the board reluctantly gave in to hiring those I had recommended, even though some were not Baptist. The Lord knew I had my bags packed so he sent me a message that said, "I put you here and you are going to stay. I'll work out these issues."

Sometimes you remember funny things that happen when under stress. In trying to save the school money, I drove down to Jefferson City to the prison to buy office furniture that the prisoners had made. Jefferson City is hilly, so to speak, down in the Ozark area. As I was driving up a hill, a couple of desks rolled off the back of the truck and went bouncing down the hill. In my mind I could just see the headlines, "Car hit by flying desk".

The next crisis came when we had to submit our
program to the State Board of Nursing. The women of
that board refused to let the program start until they
were assured the director would have full control over
the program and direct it as the state dictated.
Apparently that had been an issue between the school
and the state. In a previous attempt to start a program,
the state had denied the approval for the school's
program. One thing you must have is a good
relationship between the nursing program and the state
board of nursing. Slowly, with divine intervention, we
were able to work through these obstacles.

Six months later, a small group of citizens and Dr.
Brown accompanied me to a state board meeting, and I
presented the program and answered their questions.
The atmosphere was very warm and congenial. At the
end of the meeting I asked them if they could give us an
answer that night, which was not their policy. Usually
you had to wait for a month or so down the road. They
looked at one another, decided to vote right then, and
gave us a green light. Dr. Brown got so excited he said,
"Let's go to Dairy Queen, and I will buy you all a
milkshake!" I am sure those feminist board members
liked that idea. Now what else would you expect from a
Baptist Preacher?

Well, it was time for Ron and I to decide what we do

about my continuing with this position. So we decided to move halfway between Hannibal and St. Louis and see how that worked out for a year. Unexpectedly, his company decided to send car vans up in that area so he could just get in a van and sleep all the way to St. Louis and back. My husband can sleep anytime and anywhere. After trying that for a year, we moved to Louisiana, Missouri. Ron continued to "van it" to St. Louis and we lived there for 16 years. He became music director at the First Baptist Church in Louisiana as well. My husband was a man who respected his wife and encouraged my involvement in my profession. We were partners in our marriage and it has worked fine for us. Ron and I spent one evening burning the midnight oil with Dr. Brown and his secretary, on our knees, putting papers together to prepare our written proposal to the State Board of Nursing.

The school opened in 1981 and the first class graduated in 1983. Of course, we had to eventually seek national league accreditation, which we did in 1988. I traveled to New York to present the program to the review board and again we were able to successfully meet the standards. Prior to this time, we also developed a Bachelor of Science Completion program for Nursing. While in New York, that strange feeling came over me that indicated a change was coming. I tried to shake it off. I had a conversation with myself. "Surely the Lord would not do this to me again!'"

But before I get into that, I want to say that success came only because of submitting to The Lord and having helpers, like my fine faculty and school officials, who were able to make some concessions. The students in the program came from average families and it was enjoyable to teach them, and to see them achieve a level of success they never thought possible. It was worth all the hard work. Added blessings came as many of them went on to reach higher levels of education, go into teaching, or become nurse practitioners. What a joy to know I was able to be part of making a difference in their lives.

Since about the early nineties, the college really has come a long way. It is a good school with good people. A new president, Dr. Woody Burt, helped to make some needed changes. The student enrollment increased and more modern buildings were added. As I said, it is now a university. They started a sister college, now Southwest Baptist University, in Bolivar, Missouri. My children attended there before I ever started teaching in Hannibal.

GOD CALLING AGAIN

Having obtained national accreditation, I sensed my work there was done. Sure enough, I got a visit from the new administrator at St. Mary's Hospital. This young administrator had been brought into town to merge the two existing hospitals, and he needed a nursing person to help him with the nursing part of such a move. The other hospital was Levering Hospital. Neither he nor I realized how nearly impossible a task that would be. *I am nearing retirement, why this, Lord?*

Can you see how bringing the staffs of two rival hospitals together would not be simple? But I had seen God work before, so that gave me hope. The administrator proceeded to move rather quickly, which was to his determent. Sometimes even those who you want to follow you don't want to move that quickly. This was a tremendous change for this community.

I advised him once, "Why don't you just sit back and give the people time to absorb all of this?" I suggested that he "Be still and know that He is God." He professed to be a Christian, but he didn't seem to be familiar with that verse. He insisted on moving forward at a very rapid rate. Design for the new hospital was made and property obtained.

Opposition to all of this change was fierce. A power struggle between the administrator and the doctors rose up immediately. The two nursing staffs did not gel very easily, at first, so underlying problems arose. The nursing personnel were really good nurses, though, and in time they found a way to accept each other. The struggle between the administrator and the doctors just seemed to be one that would not or could not be resolved. Eventually the community became involved and people took sides. Of course, it was big headlines for the local newspaper.

In my opinion, mistakes were made on both sides. The good that came from it was a beautiful new, state-of-the-art hospital that now stands on the outskirts of the town. I trust at least a little credit will be given to the administrator who made this new hospital possible. My purpose in being there, at that time, I believe, was to be a calming influence amid a lot of conflict. Dr. Burt from the college told me I was a biblical Deborah. I looked up her achievements, and this is what I read: "She was known for her wisdom and courage." Well, the courage fit this situation, for sure. But I had a chuckle over this. She also was the only Hebrew woman who gained her own renown without the aid of a man. Now I did not make that up.

My husband retired and we moved to Texas to be near our new and only grandson at that time. I now would be able to plant those flowers. Although I had to discard my cap some time ago, the Diploma touch, though fading, is mine to keep and to still use in two lay ministries, one being a Stephen minister, and another a facilitator of a Grief Program. The touch keeps going on and on!

For I have plans for you, says the Lord. Plans to bless you and not to harm you, plans to give you hope and a future.
Jeremiah 29:11:

Part VII Current Status and Challenges of the Future Nurse

I do not pretend to know the future for my profession but I do believe the future will be a challenging and changing one. As of now, with the health care dispute, the end game is not decided, but it will be, and the nurse will continue to be an important player and, perhaps, have even a greater role.

My concern, though, for the present, is that the profession find a way to assure the public that clinical readiness of the graduating nursing student is resolved. Or, put it another way, have we reached the ideal method of preparing the nurse to the necessary level of clinical proficiency prior to the novice being able to function safely in a clinical setting?

I put this into a question after having interviewed recent degree nurses, and from my own observations and experience as a patient. This issue was a concern of mine even when I taught in the degree programs. A recent senior nurse student who will graduate soon expressed fear of going into the clinical setting as she did not feel clinically prepared.

Another young graduate told me that she was asked to do a procedure that she had never done and so she asked the Registered Nurse if she would do it and let her observe. Her answer was, "I will do it this time only." Many procedures cannot be learned in one observation or execution. So, this is my challenge to you who are now in nursing. Find a better and surer way of fixing this lingering issue, for the sake of the patient and the student nurse, as both deserve better. Also it will be up to the nursing profession to hold together, to see that a high quality of patient care is maintained no matter what kind of health care system becomes a reality in our country.

Even as I write, hospitals are laying off medical personnel due to the healthcare uncertainty. Will this mean the workload of those nurses who remain will be increased considerably? Doctors are threatening to quit the profession rather than to accept the new Health Care Law. Many unanswered questions abound regarding the future state of health care. We have been known as a country with the highest quality of medical and nursing care. It will be up to your generation to maintain this status.

My last word is to the hard working Licensed Practical Nurses. You have been our faithful sidekicks for many years. Your heart and touch is truly that of a nurse. You have a story to tell as well. God bless you. Never feel you were not or are not appreciated.

As Florence Nightingale so neatly expressed it, "What greater work could each of us do than to attend to those whom God puts in our path for us to display our artistry, with a touch that is creative, devoted and delicately skilled as any of the other Fine Artist."

Nursing is an art and if it is so to be made an art,
It requires as exclusive devotion, as hard a preparation
as any painter or sculptor's work;
For what is having to do with dead canvas or cold
marble,
Compared with having to do with the living body,
The temple of God's Spirit?
It is one of the Fine Arts,
I had almost said,
The finest of the Fine Arts.
Florence Nightingale

Special Recognitions

Bless you, Florence Nightingale and thank you, Alton Memorial Hospital, and all of the Registered Nurses who mentored us, and for all Diploma RNs who earned a cap and pin.

I thank my friends who encouraged me to write this story after reading some earlier attempts, namely my dear friends Mary Fleming and Mary Jane Howarth, and also Brenda Dooley and Verla Boyd, my two sisters. Thanks to Mary C. Findley, my nephew's wife, who helped edit and design this book and its cover.

Though the time frame that I focused on found an absence, or at least scarcity, of men in nursing, which I sincerely regret, I joined the ranks of those who helped make it possible for more men to be allowed to enter these programs. I admitted and taught many fine young men and they, too, became and are an asset to nursing. Florence would be proud of both her daughters and sons.

About the Author

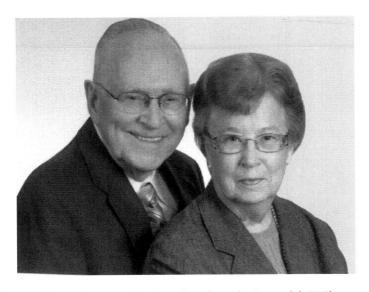

The author lives with her husband, Ronald Wilson, in Bixby, Oklahoma. They are enjoying loving on four grandchildren. Her nursing career spanned nearly forty years in nursing education and nursing administration Her passions are her family, her faith, and her profession. She had a strong desire to share what life was like as a nursing student 60 years ago, believing it would be of interest to and an inspiration for the nursing student of today. Her love for the student nurse continues to be strong. She believes they represent the best of the best.

Mrs. Wilson continues to be active in caring for hurting people. She Started a Grief Share Group Program ten years ago and is currently compiling stories about healings that she has experienced through this ministry. She and her husband are also Stephen Ministers at their church, helping individuals who are going through crises.

She feels she has had a blessed life. Her joy is to hear from former students and instructors that she taught and mentored. she hopes this story will also show her gratitude to those who gave her a start that led to a wonderful career.

PROFESSIONAL CREDENTIALS

MS in Nursing

Alton Memorial Hospital School of Nursing 1950

B.S. from Shurtleff College Alton IL 1954

MSN Washington University St. Louis University, St. Louis, MO 1957

Instructional and Administrative Career

St. Joseph and Alton Memorial Nursing Schools

Nursing Co-ordinator, Lewis and Clark Community College, 1971-1980

Director of Nursing, Hannibal La Grange College, Hannibal, MO, 1982-1988

Assistant Professor of Nursing Southern Illinois University Edwardsville IL 1966-1969

Director of Nursing St. Mary's Hospital. East St. Louis
1970-1971

Vice President of Nursing at Hannibal Regional
Hospital 1988-1991

Bibliography and Photo Credits

The Life and Work of Sigmund Freud by Ernest Jones New York: Basic Books Publishers, 1955

US Graduation Rates from High School: A Historical Review Digest of Statistics. Statistical Office of Education from Simon and Grant, 1965

Alton Evening Telegraph articles.

Hospitals, Paternalism, and the Role of the Nurse Joann Ashley Teacher's College Press Teacher's College, Columbia University, New York, New York, 1977 Second Printing

Nursing Illustrated History – The Finest Art M Patrick Donahue PhD RN CU Mosby Company St Louis Toronto Princeton 1985

Alton Memorial Hospital 75 Years of Excellence Charles Stetson Walsworth Publishing 2012

The Open Door (Nursing school Yearbook) 1950 and 1953

Max Lucado quote is from Grace for the Moment: A 365 Day Journaling Devotional Thomas Nelson; 1st

edition (June 23, 2009) HarperCollins Christian
Publishing

The Holy Bible New King James Version

Photo Credits

Images contained in the text are credited when source is
known. Image usage is included under the fair use
provision of the U.S. Copyright Law. They are small
versions of historical subjects used only to enrich a
personal memoir.

Alton historic home public domain Ralph Moran,
Wikimedia Commons

Piasa Bird Burfalcy Creative Commons

Robert Wadlow Statue Chrissy Wainwright Flicker
Creative Commons

BJC Healthcare pinterest page historic Alton Hospital
photos

Clark Bridge Alton IL Photo by Illinois2011 Wikimedia
Commons

St Mary's Catholic Church Kim Foster City Data

Studebaker Lars-Göran Lindgren Sweden Wikimedia
Commons

Florence Nightingale by Arthur George Walker, R.A.
1861-1936. 1910. Bronze. Part of the Crimean War
Memorial located facing Waterloo Place at the junction
of Lower Regent Street and Pall Mall, London.

Doctor and nurse in examining room HRC photograph collection pre 1950s.

Cadet nurses United States Government Printing Office; scan provided by Pritzker Military Library, Chicago, IL

Painting of Daughters of Charity by Karol Tichy from the National Museum in Warsaw

1947 Surgical team at Rose de Lima Hospital from the Dignity Health St. Rose Dominican website.

WWII-era bucket made by the Jonesware Metal Products Company.

Personal Photos as noted in the text

9302981R00086

Made in the USA
San Bernardino, CA
13 March 2014